Application and Review of Pediatric Pharmacotherapy

Application and Review of Pediatric Pharmacotherapy

Mark L. Glover, Pharm.D.

Associate Professor

College of Pharmacy

Nova Southeastern University

Ft. Lauderdale, Florida

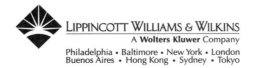

LIPPINCOTT WILLIAMS & WILKINS
A **Wolters Kluwer** Company

Philadelphia • Baltimore • New York • London
Buenos Aires • Hong Kong • Sydney • Tokyo

Senior Acquisitions Editor: David B. Troy
Managing Editor: Matthew J. Hauber
Marketing Manager: Samantha Smith
Production Editor: Jennifer P. Ajello
Designer: Risa Clow
Compositor: Graphic World
Printer: Data Reproductions Corporation

Copyright © 2004 Lippincott Williams & Wilkins
351 West Camden Street
Baltimore, MD 21201
530 Walnut Street
Philadelphia, PA 19106

Printed in the United States of America

Library of Congress Cataloging-in-Publication Data is available. ISBN: 0-7817-4253-6

The publishers have made every effort to trace the copyright holders for borrowed material. If they have inadvertently overlooked any, they will be pleased to make the necessary arrangements at the first opportunity.
To purchase additional copies of this book, call our customer service department at **(800) 638-3030** or fax orders to **(301) 824-7390.** International customers should call **(301) 714-2324.**

Visit Lippincott Williams & Wilkins on the Internet: http://www.LWW.com. Lippincott Williams & Wilkins customer service representatives are available from 8:30 am to 6:00 pm, EST.

04 05 06 07 08
1 2 3 4 5 6 7 8 9 10

This book is dedicated in memory of my father,
Joseph Clifton Glover,
and in honor of my mother,
Marjorie Murray Glover.

Preface

Medical and pharmacy students/residents often receive limited exposure to pediatric pharmacotherapy during the didactic component of their education. For this reason, their required or elective pediatric clinical rotation is often quite stressful and challenging. Additionally, the realization that providing medical care for a pediatric patient is different from caring for an adult can be intimidating to many health care professionals. Truly, pediatric patients are not merely "small adults" as they require a degree of knowledge beyond that required to provide care for the typical adult patient.

Application and Review of Pediatric Pharmacotherapy is designed as a self-assessment tool for the medical and pharmacy student/resident. Its purpose is to enhance the reader's knowledge of pediatric pharmacotherapy by allowing application of textbook information to case-based scenarios. This text is divided into four modules: Neonatal Intensive Care, Pediatric Intensive Care, Pediatric In-Patient, and Pediatric Out-Patient. Within each module there are a number of patient cases that include a medication order/prescription with an accompanying patient profile. Each of these cases is intended to mimic those that the reader may encounter as he/she is exposed to such areas of pediatrics. In many of the scenarios presented, errors have been intentionally included. Following the patient profiles

are a number of questions relating to the medication order/prescription and profile information. At the end of each section is an answer key and where appropriate, an explanation justifying the correct answer.

While this text addresses many pharmacotherapy issues relating to pediatrics, obviously some diseases are not addressed. It is the intent of this text to address the pharmacotherapy issues that are likely to be encountered during one's exposure to pediatric medicine.

Depending on the reader's level of training, some of the information and questions may seem basic. However, even the most advanced student/resident is sure to be challenged by a substantial percentage of the questions. Since this text is intended for both medical and pharmacy students/residents, some questions may be more applicable to one versus the other. Nevertheless, both parties are likely to be confronted with the information contained in each question at some point in their training or careers, and therefore are encouraged to review all the material.

Those in training and practicing pediatricians must continually review acquired knowledge and remain current on new discoveries to provide patients with optimal medical care. I trust this text will be a beneficial source for self-assessment of pediatric pharmacotherapy for those involved in the care of such patients.

Contents

Neonatal Intensive Care

*The difference between success and
failure is passion*

This section consists of 12 medication orders followed by corresponding patient profiles representing pharmacotherapy associated with patients admitted to a neonatal intensive care unit. Each patient profile is followed by multiple-choice questions pertaining to the medication order and profile information. Choose the one best-lettered response to each item. The correct answers are provided at the end of this section. The reader is encouraged to attempt all questions for each case or for the entire section prior to referring to the answer key. Moreover, where appropriate, the answer key provides a thorough explanation of the correct response and should serve as an additional learning tool for the reader.

CASE 1

PHYSICIAN ORDER

Patient Weight: 2 kg

Aminophylline 4 mg iv load, then begin 2 mg iv q 12 h
Obtain theophylline concentration 1 hour postinfusion of loading dose

Date/Time: 12/01/2100
Physician: John Craver

Patient Name: Baby Boy Turner
Patient ID #: 111222

MEDICAL PROFILE

Patient: Baby Boy Turner

Present Illness: Apneic episodes

Medical History: 33-weeks gestation, APGAR 7 and 9

Labs: Pending

Medication Profile:

Patient Weight: 2 kg   **Age:** 1 d/o

Allergies: None

1a. Which of the following is an acceptable definition of apnea of prematurity?

   A. Cessation of breathing for < 30 seconds
   B. Cessation of breathing for > 30 seconds
   C. Cessation of breathing for < 30 seconds when accompanied by bradycardia
   D. Both B and C

1b. Which of the following drug classes is represented by aminophylline?

   A. Glucocorticoid
   B. Methylxanthine
   C. Beta-adrenergic agonist
   D. Antihistamine

1c. Which is true regarding Baby Boy Turner's aminophylline regimen?

   I. The loading and maintenance doses should be increased
   II. The loading dose should be decreased
   III. The maintenance dose should be decreased

   A. I only
   B. III only
   C. I and III only
   D. II and III only
   E. I, II, and III

1d. Which of the following would be the most appropriate method of administration of Baby Boy Turner's aminophylline?

   A. An intravenous push over a 5-minute period
   B. An intravenous infusion over a 12-hour period
   C. An intravenous infusion over a 30-minute period
   D. Loading dose infused over a 5-minute period followed by the maintenance dose infused over a 12-hour period

1e. Which of the following is a potential adverse effect from aminophylline therapy?

I.   Tachycardia
II. Worsening gastroesophageal reflux
III. Agitation

    A. I only
    B. III only
    C. I and III only
    D. II and III only
    E. I, II, and III

1f. Which of the following is true regarding amino-phylline use in Baby Boy Turner?

    A. Aminophylline salt is ~ 80% theophylline
    B. Half-life is ~ 40–230 hours
    C. Therapeutic concentrations often result in urinary retention
    D. May only be diluted with normal saline

1g. As ordered, Baby Boy Turner's theophylline concentration should be approximately _____ (volume of distribution = 0.7 L/kg).

    A. 2.3 mcg/mL
    B. 2.9 mcg/mL
    C. 4.6 mcg/mL
    D. 5.7 mcg/mL

1h. Which of the following is an alternative drug that may have been prescribed to Baby Boy Turner?

I.   Caffeine
II. Doxapram
III. Oral aminophylline

    A. I only
    B. III only
    C. I and III only
    D. II and III only
    E. I, II, and III

1i. How many milliliters of a 500 mg/20 mL amino-phylline solution are required to prepare 10 mL of a 2 mg/mL dilution?

    A. 0.08 mLs
    B. 0.8 mLs
    C. 8 mLs
    D. 80 mLs

1j. The recommended therapeutic serum concentration of theophylline for patients such as Baby Boy Turner is _____.

    A. 4–12 mcg/mL
    B. 5–10 mcg/mL
    C. 5–15 mcg/mL
    D. 10–20 mcg/mL

1k. Caffeine citrate 40 mg is equivalent to _____ mg of caffeine base.

    A. 10
    B. 20
    C. 40
    D. 80

1l. Which of the following is a metabolite of theo-phylline?

I.   1-methylxanthine
II. Caffeine
III. 1- methyluric acid

    A. I only
    B. III only
    C. I and III only
    D. II and III only
    E. I, II, and III

1m. Which of the following is typically not recom-mended for neonates due to interacting competi-tively with bilirubin at albumin binding sites?

    A. Caffeine base
    B. Caffeine sodium benzoate
    C. Caffeine citrate
    D. All of the above

1n. Which of the following would be the most appro-priate loading dose of caffeine citrate for the treat-ment of apnea of prematurity?

    A. 5 mg/kg
    B. 7.5 mg/kg
    C. 20 mg/kg
    D. 30 mg/kg

CASE 2

PHYSICIAN ORDER

Patient Weight: 3 kg

Gentamicin 6 mg iv q 8 h

Date/Time: 02/21/2100
Physician: John Smith

Patient Name: Baby Boy Cooper
Patient ID #: 111211

MEDICAL PROFILE

Patient: Baby Boy Cooper

Patient Weight: 3 kg   **Age:** 1 d/o

Present Illness: R/O sepsis

Allergies: None

Medical History: 37-weeks gestation, PROM

Labs: Na 136, K 3.6, Cl 99, C02 22, Cr 0.8, BUN 6, Glu 88, WBC 10,900, H/H 10.5/30, Plat 250,000, Segs 34%, Bands 12%

Cultures: Pending

Medication Profile:

Date	Medication
2/21/2000	Ampicillin 225 mg iv q 12 h
2/21/2000	Albuterol 0.3 mg neb q 2 h
2/21/2000	Acetaminophen 30 mg po q 4 h prn

2a. The most likely pathogens present in Baby Boy Cooper would include _____.

    A. *Escherichia coli*, *Listeria* , and *Pseudomonas*
    B. *Pseudomonas*, group-B streptococci, and *Escherichia coli*
    C. *Escherichia coli*, group-B streptococci, and *Listeria*
    D. *Pseudomonas*, group-B streptococci, and *Listeria*

2b. Which of the following is a risk factor for neonatal sepsis?

    A. Premature rupture of membranes for <18 hours
    B. Prematurity
    C. High APGAR score
    D. Both A and B

2c. What is the meaning of the term "PROM"?

    A. Premature release of meconium
    B. Premature rupture of membranes
    C. Premature release of mother
    D. Premature rupture of meconium

2d. Which of the following is the most appropriate method to administer Baby Boy Cooper's ampicillin?

    A. As an infusion over a 1-hour period
    B. Via intravenous slow push
    C. Via total parenteral nutrition over a 12-hour period
    D. Via lipid emulsion over a 1-hour period

2e. Which of the following is true regarding Baby Boy Cooper's ampicillin?

A. Mechanism of action involves inhibition of protein synthesis
B. Reconstituted solution should be used within 1 hour of mixing
C. Higher doses are recommended for treating meningitis and group-B streptococcal infections
D. Both B and C

2f. Which class of drugs is represented by gentamicin?

A. Penicillins
B. Sulfonamides
C. Cephalosporins
D. Aminoglycosides

2g. Which of the following most closely resembles the mechanism of action of gentamicin on susceptible bacteria?

A. Inhibition of cell wall synthesis
B. Inhibition of protein synthesis
C. Inhibition of DNA gyrase
D. Inhibition of sterol synthesis

2h. Which of the following is true regarding Baby Boy Cooper's gentamicin?

A. May be mixed with the ampicillin prior to administration
B. Is available as a 10 mg/mL pediatric injectable solution
C. Blood sample should be stored at room temperature for several hours prior to gentamicin serum concentration being assayed
D. Should be administered via syringe pump over a 2-hour period

2i. Which of Baby Boy Cooper's medications is most likely prescribed incorrectly?

A. Ampicillin
B. Gentamicin
C. Both A and B
D. Neither A or B

2j. A gentamicin peak concentration is reported as 4 mg/L after the first dose of gentamicin. What is the approximate volume of distribution for gentamicin in Baby Boy Cooper?

A. 0.1 L/kg
B. 0.5 L/kg
C. 0.7 L/kg
D. 1.5 L/kg

2k. Which of the following is a reasonable gentamicin peak concentration for the treatment of possible sepsis in Baby Boy Cooper?

A. < 2 mcg/mL
B. 2–4 mcg/mL
C. 5–10 mcg/mL
D. 7–10 mcg/mL

2l. The elevated creatinine concentration reported in Baby Boy Cooper most likely reflects which of the following?

A. Onset of early renal failure
B. Gentamicin-induced renal failure
C. Maternal creatinine
D. Breakdown of muscle tissue

2m. Which of Baby Boy Cooper's medications may have a postantibiotic effect?

A. Gentamicin
B. Ampicillin
C. Albuterol
D. Acetaminophen

CASE 3

PHYSICIAN ORDER

Patient Weight: <u>2 kg</u>

Gentamicin 8 mg iv q 24 h
Ampicillin 50 mg iv q 6
Obtain gentamicin peak and trough with third dose

Date/Time: <u>01/21/2100</u>
Physician: <u>Joe Murphy</u>

Patient Name: <u>Baby Boy Smith</u>
Patient ID #: <u>131210</u>

MEDICAL PROFILE

Patient: Baby Boy Smith

Patient Weight: 2 kg   **Age:** 1 d/o

Present Illness: Sepsis

Allergies: None

Medical History: 35-weeks gestation, PROM, APGAR 5 and 7

Labs: Na 135, K 3.5, Cl 97, C02 21, Cr 0.2, BUN 4, Glu 76, WBC 12000, H/H 9/28, Plat 300,000, Segs 44%, Bands 15%

Blood Culture: Group-B Streptococcus

Medication Profile:

3a. Which is true regarding the ampicillin and gentamicin dosing in Baby Boy Smith?

    A. The ampicillin regimen should be adjusted
    B. The gentamicin regimen should be adjusted
    C. Neither regimen should be adjusted
    D. Both regimens should be adjusted

3b. Which of the following is synonymous with group B streptococcus?

    A. *S. pneumonia*
    B. *S. agalactiae*
    C. *S. viridans*
    D. *S. pyogenes*

3c. Which of the following lab values is consistent with Baby Boy Smith's current illness?

    A. Sodium
    B. Bands
    C. BUN
    D. Potassium

3d. Which of the following is a brand name of gentamicin?

    A. Nebcin
    B. Cytovene
    C. Geocillin
    D. Garamycin

3e. Which of the following is a brand name of ampicillin?

    A. Amoxil
    B. Omnipen
    C. Unasyn
    D. Mezlin

3f. Which of the following are available dosage forms for ampicillin?

    A. Capsules
    B. Powder for injection
    C. Powder for oral suspension
    D. A and B only
    E. A, B, and C

3g. Of the following drug classes, which most closely resembles that of ampicillin?

    A. Cephalosporins
    B. Aminoglycosides
    C. Tetracyclines
    D. Macrolides

3h. Which of the following is a major potential toxicity from gentamicin therapy?

    A. Peripheral neuropathy
    B. Nephrotoxicity
    C. Seizures
    D. Optic neuritis

3i. What would be the expected gentamicin peak concentration after Baby Boy Smith's first dose? (volume of distribution 1.2 L, half-life 6 hours)

    A. 2 mcg/mL
    B. 3.3 mg/L
    C. 6.7 mg/L
    D. 9.6 mcg/mL

3j. Gentamicin concentrations were reported as 8 mcg/mL and 1 mcg/mL at 1 and 22 hours post-third dose, respectively. What is the calculated half-life of gentamicin in Baby Boy Smith?

    A. 5 hours
    B. 7 hours
    C. 9 hours
    D. 11 hours

3k. Which of the following is not a component of the APGAR score?

    A. Activity
    B. Pulse
    C. Gestational age
    D. Appearance
    E. Respiration

3l. In preparing Baby Boy Smith's ampicillin, 10 milliliters of sterile water are added to a 1-gram vial yielding a final concentration of 1 gram per 10 milliliters. How many milliliters of this solution are needed to provide each of his prescribed doses?

    A. 0.05 mL
    B. 0.5 mL
    C. 5 mL
    D. 50 mL

3m. Which of the following bacteria is usually resistant to gentamicin?

    A. *E. coli*
    B. *Pseudomonas*
    C. *Klebsiella*
    D. MRSA

CASE 4

PHYSICIAN ORDER

Patient Weight: 3 kg

Vancomycin 30 mg iv q 12 h
Timentin 150 mg iv q 6 h

Date/Time: 05/21/2100
Physician: John Ray

Patient Name: Baby Boy Jones
Patient ID #: 213210

MEDICAL PROFILE

Patient: Baby Boy Jones

Patient Weight: 3 kg   **Age:** 7 d/o

Present Illness: Sepsis, "reactive airways"

Allergies: None

Medical History: 37-weeks gestation

Labs: Na 135, K 3.5, Cl 97, C02 21, Cr 0.2, BUN 4, Glu 76, WBC 15,000, H/H 12/36, Plat 350,000, Segs 38%, Bands 11%, CRP 8

Blood Culture: *S. epidermidis*

Medication Profile:

Date	Medication
5/21/2000	Albuterol 0.5 mg neb q 2 h
5/21/2000	Ranitidine 3mg iv q 8 h

4a. Which of the following bacteria are routinely susceptible to either of the antibiotics prescribed for Baby Boy Jones?

I. *S. aureus*
II. *S. epidermidis*
III. MRSA

    A. I only
    B. III only
    C. I and III only
    D. II and III only
    E. I, II, and III

4b. Which of the following most closely represents desired therapeutic concentrations (mcg/ml) for vancomycin?

    A. Peak 10–20, trough <5
    B. Peak 10–20, trough 5–10
    C. Peak 20–40, trough <5
    D. Peak 20–40, trough 5–10

4c. Which of the following would be a more appropriate initial vancomycin regimen for Baby Boy Jones?

    A. Vancomycin 30 mg iv q 6 h
    B. Vancomycin 60 mg iv q 6 h
    C. Vancomycin 60 mg iv q 12 h
    D. Vancomycin 30 mg iv q 8 h

4d. Which of the following is true regarding vancomycin-induced Red-man syndrome?

  A. Mechanism involves inhibition of histamine release
  B. May be minimized by infusing vancomycin over a shorter time period
  C. Vancomycin should be discontinued and alternate therapy initiated
  D. Diphenhydramine may prove beneficial if administered prior to vancomycin

4e. To prepare the dose of vancomycin, 10 mL of sterile water for injection is added to a 500 mg vial of vancomycin powder for injection yielding 500 mg/10 mL. One milliliter of this solution is added to 9 mL of sterile water to prepare the final dilution. How many milliliters should be withdrawn from this final dilution to prepare each of Baby Boy Jones' vancomycin doses?

  A. 3 mLs
  B. 5 mLs
  C. 6 mLs
  D. 7 mLs

4f. Which of the following is true regarding *S. epidermidis*?

  I. Represents a gram-positive bacteria
  II. Is a gram-negative bacteria
  III. Is often associated with intravenous catheters

    A. I only
    B. III only
    C. I and III only
    D. II and III only
    E. I, II, and III

4g. After the first dose of vancomycin, a peak concentration 1 hour postinfusion is reported as 140 mg/L. Provided a dosing error occurred, which of the following would have been most likely? (half-life = 4 hours, volume of distribution = 0.7 L/kg)

  A. A two-fold dosing error occurred
  B. A five-fold dosing error occurred
  C. A ten-fold dosing error occurred
  D. A twenty-fold dosing error occurred

4h. Which of the following is a brand name for albuterol?

  A. Proventil
  B. Serevent
  C. Intal
  D. Vanceril

4i. Which of the following most closely resembles ranitidine?

  A. Famotidine
  B. Omeprazole
  C. Metoclopramide
  D. Sucralfate

4j. Which of the following best describes the action of albuterol?

  A. α-1 agonist
  B. β-1 antagonist
  C. β-2 agonist
  D. α-2 agonist

4k. Which of the following dosage forms of vancomycin would be appropriate for Baby Boy Jones?

  A. Intravenous
  B. Oral
  C. Either oral or intravenous
  D. Rectal

4l. What does the lab "CRP" signify?

  A. C-responsive particle
  B. C-reactive protein
  C. Capillary refill pressure
  D. Carbon responsive particle

4m. Timentin is a combination of which of the following components?

  A. Ticarcillin and sulbactam
  B. Ticarcillin and clavulanic acid
  C. Ticarcillin and tazobactam
  D. Ticarcillin and ampicillin

4n. How many milligrams of ticarcillin are present in each 3.1 grams of Timentin?

  A. 100 mg
  B. 3000 mg
  C. 3100 mg
  D. 3200 mg

4o. Albuterol is available as 2.5 mg/3 mL of normal saline for nebulizer use. How many milliliters are needed to treat Baby Boy Jones for 12 hours?

  A. 3 mL
  B. 3.6 mL
  C. 6 mL
  D. 7.2 mL

4p. What is the most likely indication for ranitidine for Baby Boy Jones?

    A. Allergies
    B. Stress ulcer prophylaxis
    C. Sepsis
    D. Feeding intolerance

4q. How many milliliters of a 1 mg/mL dilution of ranitidine are necessary to provide Baby Boy Jones with his daily prescribed dose?

    A. 3 mL
    B. 6 mL
    C. 9 mL
    D. 12 mL

4r. Which additional test might be beneficial to obtain during ranitidine therapy?

    A. CBC
    B. Hematocrit
    C. Glucose
    D. Gastric pH

4s. Based on Baby Boy Jones' medical profile, which of the following medications would likely be discontinued?

    A. Vancomycin
    B. Timentin
    C. Albuterol
    D. A and B only
    E. A, B, and C

CASE 5

PHYSICIAN ORDER

Patient Weight: <u>2 kg</u>

Attempt to close PDA per protocol

Date/Time: <u>01/21/2100</u>
Physician: <u>John Sawyer</u>

Patient Name: <u>Baby Girl Smith</u>
Patient ID #: <u>211210</u>

MEDICAL PROFILE

Patient: Baby Girl Smith

Present Illness: PDA

Medical History: 34-weeks gestation

Labs: Na 135, K 3.5, Cl 97, C02 21, Cr 0.2, BUN 4, Glu 76

ABG: pH 7.32, PC02 50, P02 65, HC03 20

Medication Profile:

Patient Weight: 2 kg   **Age:** 3 d/o

Allergies: None

Date	Medication
1/20/1900	Midazolam 0.2 mg iv q 2 h prn
1/20/1900	Vecuronium 0.2 mg iv q 2 h prn

5a. Which of the following is the meaning of the term "PDA"?

   A. Patent descending aorta
   B. Paternal ductus artery
   C. Paternal descending aorta
   D. Patent ductus arteriosus

5b. Which of the following is associated with a PDA?

   I. Murmur
   II. Metabolic acidosis
   III. Widened pulse pressure

   A. I only
   B. III only
   C. I and III only
   D. II and III only
   E. I, II, and III

5c. Which of the following is true regarding a PDA?

   I. Diagnosed via echocardiogram
   II. Have been treated effectively with ibuprofen
   III. Often beneficial to patients with cyanotic congenital heart disease

   A. I only
   B. III only
   C. I and III only
   D. II and III only
   E. I, II, and III

5d. Which of the following assists in maintaining a PDA?

   A. Increased oxygenation
   B. Increased prostaglandins
   C. Decreased prostaglandins
   D. A and C

5e. Which of the following medications is most likely to be prescribed to Baby Girl Smith?

A. Phenobarbital
B. Indomethacin
C. Phenytoin
D. Alprostadil

5f. Which of the following may be prescribed to Baby Girl Smith to decrease the risk of renal dysfunction associated with the treatment of the PDA?

A. Furosemide 0.1 mg/kg
B. Furosemide 1 mg/kg
C. Sodium chloride 1 cc/kg
D. Mannitol 0.25 g/kg

5g. Which of the following is true regarding alprostadil?

A. Inhibits the release of prostaglandins
B. Administration may result in apnea for which intubation may be needed
C. A reasonable initial dose would be 0.05 mcg/kg/min
D. A and B only
E. B and C only

5h. Which of the following is true regarding indomethacin?

A. Mechanism of action involves stimulation of prostaglandin production
B. Potential adverse effects include gastrointestinal hemorrhaging and renal dysfunction
C. Is available only for oral administration
D. Maximum recommended dose is 0.2 mg every 24 hours

5i. Which of the following is a trade name for midazolam?

A. Ativan
B. Valium
C. Norcuron
D. Versed

5j. Which of the following is a trade name for vecuronium?

A. Pavulon
B. Norcuron
C. Nimbex
D. Valium

CASE 6

PHYSICIAN ORDER

Patient Weight: 1500 gms

Survanta 4.5 mLs ET q 4 h for 6 doses

Date/Time: 3/21/1000
Physician: John Parks

Patient Name: Baby Girl Thomas
Patient ID #: 215610

MEDICAL PROFILE

Patient: Baby Girl Thomas

Patient Weight: 1500 gms   **Age:** 1 d/o

Present Illness: RDS

Allergies: None

Medical History: 32-weeks gestation

Labs: Na 133, K 3.0, Cl 97, C02 24, Cr 0.1, BUN 2, Glu 80, WBC 5000, H/H 11/33, Plat 300,000, Segs 26%, Bands 3%

ABG: pH 7.30, PC02 48, P02 50, HC03 22

Medication Profile:

Date	Medication
3/21/0900	Furosemide 1.5 mg q 24 h and prn
3/21/0900	Ranitidine 1.5 mg iv q 12 h
3/21/0900	Albuterol 0.2 mg neb q 2 h

6a. Which of the following is true regarding respiratory distress syndrome?

I.   Is often referred to as hyaline membrane disease
II. Is more common in neonates > 36-weeks gestation
III. Is a consequence of surfactant deficiency

    A. I only
    B. III only
    C. I and III only
    D. II and III only
    E. I, II, and III

6b. Which of the following is associated with respiratory distress syndrome?

I.   Cyanosis
II. Oliguria
III. Edema

    A. I only
    B. III only
    C. I and III only
    D. II and III only
    E. I, II, and III

6c. Which of the following is true regarding surfactant?

   I. Is secreted primarily by type III alveolar cells

   II. Is available commercially as both natural and synthetic preparations

   III. Deficiency results in increased alveolar surface tensions, alveolar collapse, and increased work of breathing

     A. I only
     B. III only
     C. I and III only
     D. II and III only
     E. I, II, and III

6d. Which of the following route of administration is most appropriate for surfactant?

     A. Intravenous
     B. Endotracheal
     C. Oral
     D. Intramuscular

6e. Surfactant is indicated for which of the following?

   I. Prophylaxis of infants at high risk for RDS

   II. Only for infants greater than 1400 grams

   III. Rescue treatment of infants with RDS

     A. I only
     B. III only
     C. I and III only
     D. II and III only
     E. I, II, and III

6f. Which of the following is a synthetic surfactant?

     A. Exosurf
     B. Infasurf
     C. Survanta
     D. Beractant

6g. Which of the following should be modified regarding the surfactant order for Baby Girl Thomas?

   I. The dose

   II. The dosing interval

   III. The number of doses

     A. I only
     B. III only
     C. I and III only
     D. II and III only
     E. I, II, and III

6h. What is the most concerning toxicity resulting from surfactant administration?

     A. Congestive heart failure
     B. Cerebral ischemia
     C. BPD
     D. Pulmonary hemorrhaging

6i. Which of the following is true regarding Exosurf?

     A. Recommended dose is 5 mL/kg every 12 to 24 hours
     B. Is supplied as a sterile lyophilized powder necessitating refrigeration
     C. The neonate's head should remain in a midline position throughout dosing
     D. A and B only
     E. A, B, and C

6j. What is the action of the cetyl alcohol component of Exosurf?

     A. Spreading agent
     B. Preservative
     C. Solvent
     D. Nonionic lipid

6k. Which of the following is true regarding Survanta?

     A. Contains surfactant associated proteins C and D
     B. Is provided as a suspension that should be refrigerated and shaken prior to use
     C. Contains phospholipids 25 mg/mL
     D. A and C only
     E. A, B, and C

6l. Which of the following therapies would be most appropriate in an attempt to prevent RDS in a newborn?

     A. Administer nitrous oxide 4 ppm immediately after birth
     B. Extracorporeal membrane oxygenation support for 48 hours
     C. Maternal surfactant
     D. Maternal corticosteroids

6m. Which of the following medications may have influenced Baby Girl Thomas' potassium concentration?

     A. Survanta
     B. Lasix
     C. Zantac
     D. A and B only
     E. A, B, and C

CASE 7

PHYSICIAN ORDER

Patient Weight: <u>2 kg</u>

Discontinue furosemide
HCTZ 2 mg q 12 h
Spironolactone 2 mg q 12 h

Date/Time: <u>2/6/0900</u>
Physician: <u>John Quelsh</u>

Patient Name: <u>Baby Girl Daniels</u>
Patient ID #: <u>215555</u>

MEDICAL PROFILE

Patient: Baby Girl Daniels

Patient Weight: 2 kg   **Age:** 38 d/o

Present Illness: BPD, nephrocalcinosis

Allergies: None

Medical History: 33-weeks gestation, RDS, PDA

Labs: Na 132, K 2.9, Cl 96, C02 24, Cr 0.2, BUN 4, Glu 150, WBC 9000, H/H 11/33, Plat 300,000, Segs 36%, Bands 1%

ABG: pH 7.44, PC02 65, P02 59, HC03 35

Cultures: Negative

Medication Profile:

Date	Medication
2/01/1400	Furosemide 2 mg iv q 12 h
2/01/0900	Ranitidine 2 mg iv q 12 h
2/01/0900	Albuterol 0.2 mg neb q 6 h
2/01/0900	Dexamethasone 0.3 mg iv q 12 h

7a. Which of the following is associated with bronchopulmonary dysplasia (BPD)?

 I. Immature antioxidant systems
 II. Positive pressure ventilation
 III. Chronic respiratory symptoms persisting for >28 days of life

 A. I only
 B. III only
 C. I and III only
 D. II and III only
 E. I, II, and III

7b. Infants with chronic BPD typically manifest which of the following?

 A. Decreased caloric expenditure
 B. Altered gas exchange
 C. Abnormal pulmonary function
 D. B and C only
 E. A, B, and C

7c. Which of the following pathophysiologic mechanisms is associated with BPD?

   A. Pulmonary edema
   B. Airway inflammation
   C. Airway hyperreactivity
   D. A and B only
   E. A, B, and C

7d. Which of the medications prescribed to Baby Girl Daniels is most likely responsible for the nephrocalcinosis?

   A. Dexamethasone
   B. Furosemide
   C. Spironolactone
   D. Albuterol

7e. Which of the medications prescribed to Baby Girl Daniels may have influenced the reported potassium concentration?

   I. Furosemide
   II. Ranitidine
   III. Albuterol

     A. I only
     B. III only
     C. I and III only
     D. II and III only
     E. I, II, and III

7f. What dosage form of spironolactone should be prescribed for Baby Girl Daniels?

   A. Oral
   B. Intravenous
   C. Rectal
   D. Intramuscular

7g. What dosage form of hydrochlorothiazide should be prescribed for Baby Girl Daniels?

   A. Oral
   B. Intravenous
   C. Rectal
   D. Intramuscular

7h. How many milliliters of a 50 mg/5 mL commercial solution is needed to provide each dose of hydrochlorothiazide to Baby Girl Daniels?

   A. 0.2 mL
   B. 0.4 mL
   C. 2 mL
   D. 4 mL

7i. Which of the following best describes the activity of spironolactone?

   A. Loop diuretic
   B. Potassium-sparing diuretic
   C. Thiazide diuretic
   D. Carbonic anhydrase inhibitor

7j. Which of the following might benefit Baby Girl Daniels?

   I. Sodium chloride
   II. 5% Dextrose
   III. Potassium chloride

     A. I only
     B. III only
     C. I and III only
     D. II and III only
     E. I, II, and III

7k. Which of the following is a trade name for spironolactone?

   A. Aldactone
   B. Dyazide
   C. Bumex
   D. Diamox

7l. Which of the following steroids is recommended as a 42-day weaning regimen in the treatment of BPD?

   A. Methylprednisolone
   B. Dexamethasone
   C. Prednisone
   D. Hydrocortisone

7m. Which of the following may result from the use of systemic corticosteroids?

   I. Hypertension
   II. Hypokalemia
   III. Hyperglycemia

     A. I only
     B. III only
     C. I and III only
     D. II and III only
     E. I, II, and III

7n. Which of the following would be indicative of an inappropriate steroid weaning regimen?

I.   Hypoglycemia
II. Hypertension
III. Hyperglycemia

A. I only
B. III only
C. I and III only
D. II and III only
E. I, II, and III

7o. Which of the following would be the most likely explanation for Baby Girl Daniels' altered WBC?

A. Bacterial infection
B. Corticosteroid administration
C. Blood transfusions
D. Viral infection

7p. Which of the following would be the most likely consequence of Baby Girl Daniels' newly prescribed diuretic regimen?

A. Hypercalcemia, hyperkalemia, hypokalemia
B. Hypocalcemia, hyperkalemia, hypokalemia
C. Hypercalcemia, hypocalcemia, hypokalemia
D. Hypercalcemia, hypocalcemia, hyperkalemia

7q. Which of the following is true regarding Baby Girl Daniels' previous diuretic regimen?

A. The diuretic's activity is primarily focused at the distal tubule
B. The injectable formulation may also be administered orally
C. May result in a hyperchloremic alkalosis
D. A dilution prepared from stock solutions should be refrigerated until used

7r. How many milliliters of a dexamethasone 4 mg/mL stock solution are needed to prepare 20 milliliters of a 0.25 mg/mL dilution?

A. 0.8 mL
B. 1.25 mL
C. 8 mL
D. 12.5 mL

CASE 8

PHYSICIAN ORDER

Patient Weight: <u>3 kg</u>

Begin phototherapy

Date/Time: <u>11/08/1600</u>
Physician: <u>John King</u>

Patient Name: <u>Baby Girl Parokas</u>
Patient ID #: <u>215444</u>

MEDICAL PROFILE

Patient: Baby Girl Parokas

Patient Weight: 3 kg   **Age:** 2 d/o

Present Illness: Hyperbilirubinemia

Allergies: None

Medical History: 36-weeks gestation

Labs: Na 135, K 3.6, Cl 100, C02 24, Cr 0.2, BUN 2, Glu 86, WBC 5000, H/H 11/33, Plat 300,000, Segs 36%, Bands 1%, D Bili 4, I Bili 17, Alb 3

Cultures: Negative

Medication Profile:

Date	Medication
11/8/0900	Bactrim 15 mg iv q 12 h
11/8/0900	Furosemide 3 mg iv prn
11/8/0900	Ampicillin 300 mg iv q 12 h
11/8/0900	Gentamicin 12 mg iv q 24 h

8a. Which of the following terms refers to the yellow staining of the basal ganglia observed in infants with severe jaundice?

   A. Hyperbilirubinemia
   B. Kernicterus
   C. Neonatal jaundice
   D. Hyperbiliverdin

8b. Which of the following accounts for most cases of pathologic jaundice in newborns?

   I. Impaired conjugation of bilirubin
   II. Decreased enterohepatic circulation of bilirubin
   III. Increased bilirubin production

   A. I only
   B. III only
   C. I and III only
   D. II and III only
   E. I, II, and III

8c. Which of the following is an immediate precursor to bilirubin?

A. Heme
B. Hemoglobin
C. Carboxyhemoglobin
D. Biliverdin

8d. What is Baby Girl Parokas' total bilirubin concentration?

A. 13 mg/dL
B. 17 mg/dL
C. 21 mg/dL
D. 24 mg/dL

8e. What would be the approximate maximum serum concentration of albumin-bound bilirubin in Baby Girl Parokas?

A. 10 mg/dL
B. 20 mg/dL
C. 25 mg/dL
D. 30 mg/dL

8f. Which of the following facilitates the entry of bilirubin into the brain?

A. Increased binding of bilirubin to albumin
B. Conjugation of bilirubin
C. Damaged blood-brain barrier
D. Increased oxyhemoglobin

8g. Which of Baby Girl Parokas' medications has been implicated in increasing the risk of kernicterus?

A. Bactrim
B. Furosemide
C. Ampicillin
D. Gentamicin

8h. Which of the following medications might prove useful in treating hyperbilirubinemia?

A. Phenytoin
B. Phenobarbital
C. Valproic acid
D. Dexamethasone

8i. Bactrim is a combination product consisting of trimethoprim and _____.

A. sulfamethoxazole
B. sulfisoxazole
C. sulfadiazine
D. sulfacetamide

8j. Which of the following products contains the same active ingredients as Bactrim?

A. Septra
B. Gantanol
C. Zosyn
D. Gantrisin

8k. By convention, Bactrim is dosed according to the trimethoprim component. How many milliliters of injectable Bactrim (trimethoprim 80 mg/5 mL) are needed to provide Baby Girl Parokas with her daily dose?

A. 0.5 mL
B. 0.9 mL
C. 1.5 mL
D. 1.9 mL

8l. Which of the following should not be prescribed to Baby Girl Parokas?

A. Normal saline
B. Dextrose 5%
C. Lactated ringers
D. Benzyl alcohol

CASE 9

PHYSICIAN ORDER

Patient Weight: 3.5 kg

Enalaprilat 20 mcg iv q 6 h

Date/Time: 12/09/1700
Physician: John Steeps

Patient Name: Baby Girl Prince
Patient ID #: 223444

MEDICAL PROFILE

Patient: Baby Girl Prince

Patient Weight: 3.5 kg   **Age:** 7 d/o

Present Illness: Hypertension (B/P 100/74), bronchospasms   **Allergies:** None

Medical History: 40-weeks gestation

Labs: Na 134, K 3.2, Cl 100, C02 24, Cr 0.2, BUN 2, Glu 86

Medication Profile:

Date	Medication
12/7/0900	Chlorothiazide 20 mg po q 12 h
12/7/0900	Albuterol 0.5 mg neb q 4 h
12/8/0500	Potassium chloride 1 mEq po q 8 h

9a.   Enalaprilat is an example of what class of medications?

   A.   Calcium-channel blocker
   B.   Thiazide diuretic
   C.   Angiotensin-converting enzyme inhibitor
   D.   β-adrenergic blocker

9b.   The brand name for chlorothiazide is _____.

   A.   Hydrodiuril
   B.   Diuril
   C.   Enduron
   D.   Dyazide

9c.   Baby Girl Prince's reported potassium concentration is most likely the result of which medication?

   A.   Chlorothiazide
   B.   Albuterol
   C.   Enalaprilat
   D.   A and B only
   E.   A, B, and C

9d.   Which of the following is likely to result from the administration of chlorothiazide?

   A.   Hypoglycemia
   B.   Hyperkalemia
   C.   Hyperuricemia
   D.   Hypocalcemia

9e. Which of the following is true regarding the pre-scribed regimen of enalaprilat for Baby Girl Prince?

   A. Is appropriate as prescribed
   B. The dosing interval should be modified
   C. The dose should be modified
   D. Should be dosed in milligrams instead of mi-crograms

9f. Which of the following medications most closely resembles enalaprilat?

   A. Chlorothiazide
   B. Captopril
   C. Atenolol
   D. Verapamil

9g. Which of the following is true regarding Baby Girl Prince's chlorothiazide?

   A. Should be dosed every 6 hours initially
   B. Should be dosed 10–20 mg/kg/dose
   C. Is only available as an oral preparation
   D. Is classified as a loop diuretic

9h. Which of the following is true regarding enalaprilat?

   A. Is available as a 1.50 mg/mL stock solution
   B. Is hydrolyzed in the liver to the active drug, enalapril
   C. Is contraindicated in the presence of bilateral renal artery stenosis
   D. Often requires coadministration of potassium chloride

9i. The prescribing of chlorothiazide to Baby Girl Prince was most likely an effort to achieve which of the following?

   A. Normalize her serum potassium concentration
   B. Antagonize the cardiovascular effects of al-buterol
   C. Allow for discontinuation of potassium chloride
   D. Further reduce the blood pressure by providing another mechanism of action

9j. Which of the following is true regarding Baby Girl Prince's prescribed potassium chloride?

   A. Should not be diluted prior to administration
   B. Preferably should be administered intravenously
   C. May result in gastric irritation
   D. Should only be dosed in milligrams

CASE 10

PHYSICIAN ORDER

Patient Weight: <u>1200 gms</u>

Phenobarbital 5 mg/kg loading dose followed by
1 mg/kg/day for 4 days

Date/Time: <u>4/6/0900</u>
Physician: <u>David Ostey</u>

Patient Name: <u>Baby Boy Spree</u>
Patient ID #: <u>215665</u>

MEDICAL PROFILE

Patient: Baby Boy Spree

Patient Weight: 1200 gms   **Age:** 1 d/o

Present Illness: IVH, R/O sepsis

Allergies: None

Medical History: 32-weeks gestation

Labs: Na 138, K 3.8, Cl 102, C02 22, Cr 0.6, BUN 4, Glu 98, WBC 4000, H/H 12/36, Plat 300,000, Segs 33%, Bands 2%

ABG: pH 7.42, PC02 59, P02 39, HC03 21

Cultures: Pending

Medication Profile:

Date	Medication
4/6/0200	Gentamicin 5 mg iv qd
4/6/0200	Ampicillin 125 mg iv q 12
4/6/0200	Vecuronium 0.12 mg iv q 1 h prn
4/6/0200	Midazolam 0.12 mg iv q 2 h prn

10a. Which of the following is a risk factor for intraventricular hemorrhaging (IVH)?

   A. Less than 34-weeks gestation
   B. Birthweight > 1500 grams
   C. Use of sedative agents
   D. A and B only
   E. A, B, and C

10b. Which of the following might serve as a useful indication of IVH?

   A. Failure to thrive
   B. Poor feeding
   C. Unexplained fall in hematocrit
   D. Fever

10c. According to the Papile IVH grading system, which grade is defined as IVH with ventricular dilatation?

A. I
B. II
C. III
D. IV

10d. According to the Papile IVH grading system, which grade is often associated with at least a 50% frequency of mental and/or motor handicaps?

A. I
B. II
C. III
D. IV

10e. Which of the following is a potential consequence of IVH?

A. Seizures
B. Hydrocephalus
C. Hemorrhagic infarction
D. A and B only
E. A, B, and C

10f. For optimal response in preventing IVH, pharmacotherapy should be initiated within _____ hours of birth.

A. 3
B. 6
C. 9
D. 12

10g. Which of the following would be a reasonable alternative to phenobarbital for Baby Boy Spree?

A. Phenytoin
B. Valproic acid
C. Midazolam
D. Indomethacin

10h. Which of the following are potential benefits from phenobarbital therapy for Baby Boy Spree?

A. Increase cerebral blood flow
B. Increase catecholamine release
C. Blunt swings in blood pressure
D. Increase cerebral metabolic rate

10i. Which of the following is true regarding Baby Boy Spree's phenobarbital regimen?

A. Is appropriate as prescribed
B. Should be 5 mg/kg loading dose, then 5 mg/kg/day for 4 days
C. Should be 20 mg/kg loading dose, then 5 mg/kg/day for 4 days
D. Omit loading dose and prescribe 5 mg/kg/day for 4 days

10j. In preparing Baby Boy Spree's phenobarbital loading dose as prescribed, which of the following would be most appropriate?

A. Use a 65 mg/mL stock solution
B. Use a 130 mg/mL stock solution
C. Prepare a 10 mg/mL dilution
D. Prepare a 100 mg/mL dilution

10k. Vecuronium is classified as a(n)

_____.

A. nondepolarizing neuromuscular blocking agent
B. depolarizing neuromuscular blocking agent
C. benzodiazepine
D. opiate

10l. Which of Baby Boy Spree's medications might increase the potential adverse effects from vecuronium therapy?

A. Gentamicin
B. Dexamethasone
C. Ampicillin
D. Midazolam

10m. Which of the following is a reasonable targeted phenobarbital concentration for Baby Boy Spree?

A. 5–15 mcg/mL
B. 10–20 mcg/mL
C. 15–40 mcg/mL
D. 40–60 mg/L

10n. Which of the following is an appropriate technique to initiate in patients at risk for IVH?

A. Avoid increases in cerebral blood flow
B. Minimize acute changes in arterial blood pressure
C. Minimize coagulation complications
D. A and B only
E. A, B, and C

CASE 11

PHYSICIAN ORDER

Patient Weight: <u>3 kg</u>

Increase fentanyl to 8 mcg/kg/hr

Date/Time: <u>5/21/0700</u>
Physician: <u>Trent Phillips</u>

Patient Name: <u>Baby Boy Carl</u>
Patient ID #: <u>325665</u>

MEDICAL PROFILE

Patient: Baby Boy Carl

Patient Weight: 3 kg   **Age:** 2 d/o

Present Illness: PPHN, ECMO support

Allergies: None

Medical History: 37-weeks gestation

Labs: Na 140, K 3.7, Cl 102, C02 19, Cr 0.4, BUN 2, Glu 89, WBC 6000, H/H 12/36, Plat 350,000, Segs 27%, Bands 4%, ACT 190, PT 11, PTT 70

Cultures: Pending

Medication Profile:

Date	Medication
5/20/2200	Cefotaxime 150 mg iv q 8 h
5/20/2200	Ampicillin 300 mg iv q 12 h
5/20/2300	Dopamine 10 mg/kg/min
5/21/0100	Vecuronium 0.1 mg/kg/hr
5/21/0100	Lorazepam 0.1 mg/kg/hr
5/21/0100	Fentanyl 18 mcg/hr
5/21/0300	Heparin 25 u/kg/min

11a. Which of the following indicates Baby Boy Carl's present illness?

 A. Persistent pulmonary hypertension
 B. Persistent fetal circulation
 C. Prenatal hypertension
 D. A and B only
 E. A, B, and C

11b. Which of the following is true regarding PPHN?

 A. Results in excessive blood being shunted to the lungs
 B. Results in hypoxemia with consequent vaso-constriction
 C. Treatment options include ECMO and/or nitric oxide
 D. B and C only
 E. A, B, and C

11c. The acronym "ECMO" represents
_____.

    A. external circulation membrane oxygenation
    B. extracorporeal membrane oxygenation
    C. external circulation maximal oxygenation
    D. endocorporeal maximal oxygenation

11d. Which of the following is true regarding ECMO?

    A. Is essentially heart-lung bypass of the newborn
    B. Is contraindicated in the presence of heparin administration
    C. May alter the pharmacokinetics/pharmacodynamics of select drugs
    D. A and C only
    E. B and C only

11e. Which of the following is a component of an ECMO circuit?

    A. Venoarterial or venovenous connection
    B. Membrane oxygenator
    C. Roller pump
    D. A and B only
    E. A, B, and C

11f. What is the most likely reason for increasing the fentanyl dose in Baby Boy Carl?

    A. Previous prescribed dose was lower than the "normal" therapeutic dose
    B. Higher dose needed as a result of drug being removed by the ECMO circuit
    C. Higher doses are often needed when combined with lorazepam therapy
    D. Dopamine increases fentanyl clearance necessitating higher doses

11g. Which of the following is true regarding nitric oxide?

    A. Also known as endothelium-derived relaxing factor
    B. Exerts its effects by activation of cyclic AMP
    C. Is also known as "laughing gas"
    D. A and B only
    E. A, B, and C

11h. Due to potential toxicity, which of the following should be carefully monitored during nitric oxide administration?

    A. Cyclic AMP
    B. Cyclic GMP
    C. Methemoglobin
    D. Heme

11i. Which of the following would represent a reasonable prescribed dose of nitric oxide?

    A. 20 mg
    B. 20 mcg
    C. 20 ng
    D. 20 ppm

11j. The lab value "ACT" refers to _____.

    A. actual clotting time
    B. activated clotting time
    C. accurate clotting test
    D. actual coagulation time

11k. ACT values are being obtained to monitor the effects of which of Baby Boy Carl's medications?

    A. Dopamine
    B. Heparin
    C. Fentanyl
    D. Vecuronium

11l. Which of Baby Boy Carl's medications is incorrectly prescribed?

    A. Cefotaxime
    B. Lorazepam
    C. Fentanyl
    D. Dopamine

11m. Baby Boy Carl's heparin dosage should be modified to _____.

    A. 25 mg/kg/min
    B. 25 u/kg/hr
    C. 25 mcg/kg/hr
    D. 25 mg/kg/min

CASE 12

PHYSICIAN ORDER

Patient Weight: 3 kg

AZT 3 mg po q 12 h

Date/Time: 4/12/2100
Physician: Don Little

Patient Name: Baby Boy Harris
Patient ID #: 665222

MEDICAL PROFILE

Patient: Baby Boy Harris

Patient Weight: 3 kg   **Age:** 1 d/o

Present Illness: R/O sepsis

Allergies: None

Medical History: 38-weeks gestation, mother HIV positive

Labs: Na 138, K 3.6, Cl 109, CO2 20, Cr 0.6, BUN 4, Glu 98, WBC 8000, H/H 11/33, Plat 325,000, Segs 35%, Bands 10%

Cultures: Pending

Medication Profile:

Date	Medication
4/12/1500	Cefotaxime 50 mg iv q 6 h
4/12/1500	Ampicillin 300 mg iv q 12 h

12a. Cefotaxime is marketed as _____.

A. Claforan
B. Rocephin
C. Fortaz
D. Ceftin

12b. Cefotaxime is classified as a _____ generation cephalosporin.

A. first
B. second
C. third
D. fourth

12c. A more appropriate cefotaxime regimen for Baby Boy Harris would be _____.

A. 150 mg iv q 8 h
B. 150 mg iv q 6 h
C. 300 mg iv q 12 h
D. 300 mg iv q 8 h

12d. Which of the following is true regarding the transmission of HIV from mother to fetus/infant?

A. The majority of transmission occurs around the time of delivery
B. The risk of transmission is increased for breast-feeding mothers
C. A healthy placenta protects the fetus in utero for most of gestation
D. A and B only
E. A, B, and C

12e. AZT is also known as _____.

    A. retrovir
    B. azidothymidine
    C. 3TC
    D. A and B only
    E. A, B, and C

12f. AZT is classified as a _____.

    A. protease inhibitor
    B. nucleoside reverse transcriptase inhibitor
    C. non-nucleoside reverse transcriptase inhibitor
    D. DNA polymer inhibitor

12g. During labor and delivery, Baby Boy Harris' mother most likely received which of the following AZT regimens?

    A. An infusion of 1 mg/kg/hr
    B. An infusion of 2 mg/kg/hr
    C. 1 mg/kg loading dose followed by an infusion of 1 mg/kg/hr
    D. 2 mg/kg loading dose followed by an infusion of 1 mg/kg/hr

12h. A more appropriate AZT regimen for Baby Boy Harris would be _____.

    A. 3 mg po q 8 h
    B. 3 mg po q 6 h
    C. 6 mg po q 8 h
    D. 6 mg po q 6 h

12i. AZT therapy should be initiated in Baby Boy Harris within _____ hours of birth.

    A. 12
    B. 24
    C. 36
    D. 48

12j. Baby Boy Harris should receive AZT therapy for at least _____ weeks.

    A. 4
    B. 6
    C. 8
    D. 12

MODULE 1 ANSWERS

CASE 1

1a. (D) Apnea of prematurity is often defined as cessation of breathing for > 30 seconds or < 30 seconds when accompanied by bradycardia.

1b. (B) Aminophylline, theophylline, and caffeine are methylxanthines.

1c. (A) There is an increased volume of distribution (~0.7–1 L/kg) for theophylline in preterm neonates compared with children and adults. Therefore, a higher loading dose (aminophylline 8–10 mg/kg) would be more appropriate, especially if an initial higher theophylline serum concentration is desired. A reasonable initial maintenance dose would be 2.5 mg/kg q 12 h. Therefore, a reasonable initial aminophylline regimen for Baby Boy Turner would be a loading dose of 16–20 mg (8–10 mg/kg) and a maintenance dose of 5 mg iv q 12 h (2.5 mg/kg × 2 kg = 5 mg).

1d. (C) Intravenous aminophylline is most often administered as a 30-minute infusion.

1e. (E) Potential adverse effects of aminophylline include stimulation of the central nervous system and cardiovascular system. It also decreases lower esophageal sphincter pressure that may aggravate gastroesophageal reflux.

1f. (A) Aminophylline salt is ~ 80% theophylline. The half-life in neonates is ~ 30–40 hours. Diuresis is a potential effect of all methylxanthines, including aminophylline. Aminophylline may be diluted in normal saline or 5% dextrose.

1g. (A) To estimate the concentration post-loading dose, the equation, Concentration = Dose/Volume of Distribution, may be used. Since aminophylline is 80% theophylline, a 4-mg dose of aminophylline equals 3.2 mg of theophylline (4 mg × 0.8 (80% theophylline) = 3.2 mg theophylline). For the units to cancel, the dose may be expressed in mg/kg. Therefore, 3.2 mg/2 kg = 1.6 mg/kg. So, Concentration = 1.6 mg/kg / 0.7 L/kg = 2.3 mg/L or mcg/mL.

1h. (E) Caffeine is another methylxanthine that is often prescribed for apnea of prematurity. Although not as well studied, doxapram is a non-methylxanthine alternative; however, it does contain a large amount of benzyl alcohol. Adverse effects include hypertension, abdominal distention, and central nervous system stimulation. Initial loading and maintenance doses are 3 mg/kg and 1 mg/kg/hr, respectively. Oral aminophylline may have also been prescribed.

1i. (B) To prepare 10 mLs of a 2 mg/mL dilution, 20 mg are needed (10 mLs × 2 mg/mL = 20 mg). Therefore, 500 mg/20 mL = 20 mg/x; x = 0.8 mL.

1j. (C)

1k. (B) Caffeine citrate is 50% caffeine base. Caffeine citrate 40 mg × 0.5 (50%) = 20 mg caffeine base.

1l. (E) 1-methylxanthine and 1-methyluric acid are metabolites of theophylline in both children and adults. Caffeine is a theophylline metabolite during the neonatal period.

1m. (B) Caffeine sodium benzoate may result in increased free bilirubin concentrations due to competitively interacting at the albumin binding sites, thus possibly leading to kernicterus.

1n. (C) Caffeine citrate 20 mg/kg = caffeine base 10 mg/kg; an appropriate loading dose for an initial concentration of ~ 10–15 mg/L.

CASE 2

2a. (C) The most common bacterial pathogens in newborns are group-B streptococcus, *E. coli*, and *Listeria*.

2b. (B) Risk factors for neonatal sepsis include premature rupture of membranes (PROM) for > 18 hours, low APGAR scores, maternal fever, maternal colonization with group-B streptococcus, and prematurity.

2c. (B)

2d. (B) Ampicillin is most often administered over a few minutes via intravenous slow push.

2e. (D) Ampicillin's mechanism of action involves inhibition of bacterial cell wall synthesis. Because of loss of potency, reconstituted solutions should be used within 1 hour. Higher doses (i.e., 100 mg/kg) are recommended for meningitis and group-B streptococcal infections.

2f. (D)

2g. (B) Aminoglycosides, such as gentamicin, bind to the bacteria's 30S ribosome, thus inhibiting bacterial protein synthesis resulting in bacterial cell death.

2h. (B) Inactivation of gentamicin by penicillins appears to be time-, temperature-, and concentration-dependent. It may be clinically relevant if gentamicin is mixed with penicillins or if a blood sample is allowed to remain at room temperature several hours prior to assaying the serum drug concentration. Gentamicin is routinely administered via syringe pump as a 30-minute infusion. It is available as a 10 mg/mL pediatric injectable solution.

2i. (B) The volume of distribution of gentamicin approximates that of extracellular fluid (ECF). In the newborn, ECF, as a percentage of total body weight, is increased compared with children and adults. Also, gentamicin is eliminated by the kidneys via glomerular filtration. Since the glomerular filtration rate (GFR) is decreased in newborns, the clearance of gentamicin is diminished. Based on these gentamicin pharmacokinetics in newborns (volume of distribution = ~0.5 L/kg, half-life = ~6 hours), it should be dosed at a higher mg/kg dose (~ 4–5 mg/kg) and administered less frequently (q 24–48 hours). Therefore, a more appropriate initial gentamicin regimen for Baby Boy Cooper would be 12 mg (4 mg/kg × 3 kg = 12 mg) iv q 24 hours with further dosage adjustments based on serum gentamicin concentrations obtained. Dosing ampicillin at 50–100 mg/kg every 12 hours is appropriate. Baby Boy Cooper is receiving 75 mg/kg/dose of ampicillin (225 mg/3 kg = 75 mg/kg).

2j. (B) After an initial dose of gentamicin in Baby Boy Cooper, the volume of distribution can be approximated by the equation, Volume of Distribution = Dose/Concentration. Therefore, volume of distribution = 6 mg/4 mg/L = 1.5 L or 0.5 L/kg (1.5 L/3 kg = 0.5 L/kg).

2k. (D)

2l. (C) A newborn's serum creatinine is often elevated for several days (typically 3–4 days) after birth reflecting maternal creatinine. Having only received one or two doses of gentamicin, drug-induced renal dysfunction would be unlikely.

2m. (A) The aminoglycosides (i.e., gentamicin) exhibit a postantibiotic effect of which refers to the persistence of antibacterial activity in the presence of minimal serum drug concentrations.

CASE 3

3a. (A) A reasonable ampicillin regimen for a newborn such as Baby Boy Smith (35-weeks gestation, 1 day old) would be 50–100 mg/kg q 12 hours.

3b. (B) Group-B streptococcus is also known as *Streptococcus agalactiae*.

3c. (B) In response to sepsis, increased numbers of immature white blood cells are often released from the bone marrow resulting in an increase in the percentage of reported "bands," also referred to as a "left shift."

3d. (D) The respective brand and generic drug names are: Nebcin (tobramycin), Cytovene (ganciclovir), Geocillin (carbenicillin), and Garamycin (gentamicin).

3e. (B) The respective brand and generic drug names are: Amoxil (amoxicillin), Omnipen (ampicillin), Unasyn (ampicillin and sulbactam), Mezlin (mezlocillin).

3f. (E)

3g. (A) Ampicillin is an example of a penicillin. A beta-lactam ring is present in the chemical structure of both penicillins and cephalosporins.

3h. (B) The major toxicities of the aminoglycosides (i.e., gentamicin) are ototoxicity and nephrotoxicity.

3i. (C) The peak gentamicin concentration after the first dose can be estimated by the equation: Concentration = Dose/Volume of Distribution. Therefore, Concentration = 8 mg/1.2 L = 6.7 mg/L.

3j. (B) A half-life of a drug is the time required for the concentration to decrease by one-half. In this example, the gentamicin concentration decreased from 8 mcg/mL to 1 mcg/mL in 21 hours (the time difference between 1- and 22-hours postdose). Further, a decrease from 8 mcg/mL to 1 mcg/mL indicates the concentration decreased by one-half 3 times (8–4 mcg/mL, 4–2 mcg/mL, and 2–1mcg/mL) representing three half-lives. Therefore, if 21 hours represents three half-lives, then one half-life is 7 hours (21 hrs/3 half-lives = 7 hrs/half-life).

3k. (C) APGAR score is based on activity (muscle tone), pulse, grimace, appearance, and respiration. A maximum of two points is permitted for each sign with the maximum achievable score being ten. Newborns are typically scored twice, at 1 and 5 minutes after birth.

3l. (B) One gram per 10 mL = 1000 mg/10 mL or 100 mg/mL. Baby Boy Smith's dose is 50 mg. Therefore, 1000 mg/10 mL = 50 mg/x; x = 0.5 mL.

3m. (D) Gentamicin is an aminoglycoside antibiotic generally prescribed to treat gram-negative aerobic bacteria. *E. coli*, *Pseudomonas*, and *Klebsiella* are gram- negative bacteria that are typically sensitive to gentamicin. MRSA is methicillin- resistant *Staphylococcus aureus*, a gram-positive bacteria.

CASE 4

4a. (E) Vancomycin is generally prescribed to treat gram-positive bacteria. Therefore, gram-positive bacteria such as *S. aureus*, *S. epidermidis*, and MRSA are usually sensitive to vancomycin.

4b. (D) In the absence of treating highly invasive infections such as meningitis, many clinicians only monitor vancomycin trough concentrations and usually target serum concentrations of 5–10 mcg/mL. When peak concentrations are obtained, a target of 20–40 mcg/mL is acceptable with concentrations in the upper limit usually indicated for the more invasive infections.

4c. (C) In the presence of "normal" renal function, a reasonable initial vancomycin regimen for a 37-week gestation newborn, such as Baby Boy Jones, would be 20 mg/kg q 12 hours (20 mg/kg × 3 kg = 60 mg iv q 12 h). In the presence of renal dysfunction, an initial dose of 20 mg/kg may be given with concentrations obtained on the initial dose for use in performing a pharmacokinetic analysis to define an appropriate regimen.

4d. (D) Red-man syndrome is an infusion-related adverse effect of vancomycin therapy due to the release of histamine. Patients exhibiting Red-man syndrome should not be labeled as "allergic" to vancomycin as such a notation in their medical record may prevent them from receiving future therapy when indicated. Extending the infusion time of vancomycin (i.e., 2-hour infusion) and/or administering an antihistamine, such as diphenhydramine (Benadryl), may reduce the occurrence of the reaction.

4e. (C) A 500-mg vial of vancomycin reconstituted with 10 mL of sterile water yields 500 mg/10 mL or 50 mg/mL. Diluting 1 mL (50 mg) of this solution with 9 mL of sterile water = 50 mg/10 mL (1 mL of solution + 9 mL of water) or 5 mg/mL. In preparing Baby Boy Jones' prescribed dose of 30mg; 5 mg/mL = 30 mg/x; x = 6 mLs.

4f. (C) *S. epidermidis* is a gram-positive bacteria that is often suspected in potentially septic hospitalized patients in whom intravenous catheters have been placed.

4g. (C) Several possibilities for the elevated vancomycin concentration should be explored. Those would include proper timing of the blood sample, proper flushing of the intravenous line prior to obtaining

the blood sample, and proper administration of the drug. To explore the possibility of a dosing error, a vancomycin dose of 10 mg/kg (30 mg/3 kg = 10 mg/kg) should result in an initial concentration of ~ 14 mg/L (Concentration = Dose/Volume of Distribution; Concentration = 10 mg/kg/0.7 L/kg = 14.3 mg/L). Therefore, the concentration of 140 mcg/mL reported in Baby Boy Jones would indicate a 10-fold overdose (14 mg/L × 10 = 140 mg/L). A follow-up vancomycin concentration should be obtained to authenticate the initial concentration and to guide further dosing.

4h. (A) The respective brand and generic names are as follows: Proventil and Ventolin (albuterol), Serevent (salmeterol), Intal (cromolyn), Vanceril (beclomethasone).

4i. (A) Like ranitidine (Zantac), famotidine (Pepcid) is another histamine-2 antagonist.

4j. (C) Albuterol is a selective β-2 agonist that activates adenyl cyclase to produce cyclic adenosine monophosphate (cAMP), which activates various proteins by cAMP dependent protein kinase resulting in decreased unbound intracellular calcium producing smooth muscle relaxation. At high doses, the beta selectively may be compromised with β-1 agonist activity being manifested.

4k. (A) Although vancomycin is available in both parenteral and oral dosage forms, only the parenteral dosage form is indicated for systemic infections. The oral dosage form is indicated for the treatment of gastrointestinal Clostridium difficile. Because of the emergence of vancomycin resistance (i.e., vancomycin-resistant enterococci [VRE]), institutional guidelines should be followed closely regarding the appropriate use of vancomycin.

4l. (B) CRP (C-Reactive Protein) is an acute phase reactant that is often elevated in the presence of a bacterial infection. Normal values are usually < 1 mg/dL.

4m. (B)

4n. (B) Timentin 3.1 gms consist of 3000 mg of ticarcillin and 100 mg of clavulanic acid. The dose is based on the ticarcillin component of Timentin.

4o. (B) For Baby Boy Jones, 6 doses are needed in 12 hours (every 2-hour dosing). Therefore, 6 doses × 0.5 mg/dose = 3 mg. Therefore, 2.5 mg/3 mL = 3 mg/x; x = 3.6 mL.

4p. (B) Intensive care patients are often prescribed medications for stress ulcer prophylaxis with the H_2

antagonists (i.e., ranitidine) being commonly used. In the presence of a coagulopathy or respiratory failure, prophylaxis is warranted. The necessity for prophylaxis under other conditions is less clear. Given Baby Boy Jones' profile, the use of ranitidine could be questioned.

4q. (C) Baby Boy Jones' daily dose of ranitidine = 9 mg (3 mg three times a day). Therefore, 1 mg/ mL = 9 mg/x; x = 9 mL.

4r. (D) H_2 antagonists, such as ranitidine (Zantac) alter the pH of the stomach from its normal acidic to a more alkaline environment. In a patient with an existing nasogastric tube, obtaining a gastric aspirate and assessing pH values may assist in adjusting the dose based on desired pH values.

4s. (B) With a culture reported positive for *S. epidermidis*, vancomycin alone should be adequate coverage. Therefore, the clinician may wish to discontinue Timentin therapy.

CASE 5

5a. (D) The ductus arteriosus (DA) is a normal fetal vascular connection between the left pulmonary artery and the descending aorta that, in utero, allows the majority of blood flow leaving the right ventricle to circumvent the pulmonary circulation and flow directly into the descending aorta. This allows oxygen-deprived blood to flow to the placenta, the fetal source of oxygenation. After birth, the closure of the DA is usually spontaneous allowing blood to be redirected to the lungs for oxygenation. A DA that does not close is referred to as a patent ductus arteriosus (PDA).

5b. (E) Typical signs of a PDA include a murmur, bounding peripheral pulses, widened pulse pressure, tachypnea, tachycardia, edema, metabolic acidosis, and enlarged heart.

5c. (E) A PDA is diagnosed with the aid of an echocardiogram indicating a left to right shunt and increased left atrium to aorta ratio. Patients with cyanotic congenital heart disease (hypoplastic left heart, tricuspid atresia) benefit from a PDA that should be maintained with the administration of prostaglandin until corrective surgery is performed. Intravenous ibuprofen has been shown to be as effective as indomethacin for the closure of a PDA.

5d. (B) Increased oxygen tension and decreased prostaglandins act to close the ductus arteriosus. Increased prostaglandin concentrations promote patency of the ductus.

5e. (B) Indomethacin is a prostaglandin inhibitor that will act to close the ductus arteriosus.

5f. (B) Furosemide (Lasix) has been shown to reduce the risk of nephrotoxicity induced by indomethacin. A reasonable dose would be 1 mg/kg with each dose of indomethacin.

5g. (E) Alprostadil is a prostaglandin preparation used to maintain the patency of the ductus arteriosus. Administration may result in apnea. It is typically dosed between 0.025–0.4 mcg/kg/min.

5h. (B) Indomethacin is a prostaglandin inhibitor available in both oral and parenteral dosage forms. A typical dose is 0.1–0.25 mg/kg every 12 hours. Adverse effects include gastrointestinal hemorrhaging and renal dysfunction.

5i. (D) The respective trade and generic names are: Ativan (lorazepam), Valium (diazepam), Norcuron (vecuronium), and Versed (midazolam).

5j. (B) The respective trade and generic names are: Pavulon (pancuronium), Norcuron (vecuronium), Nimbex (cisatracurium), and Valium (diazepam).

CASE 6

6a. (C) Respiratory distress syndrome (RDS), also known as hyaline membrane disease, is a consequence of surfactant deficiency and is more common in neonates < 36-weeks gestation.

6b. (E) Signs of RDS include respiratory distress, cyanosis, fluid retention, and oliguria.

6c. (D) Surfactant is secreted by type II pneumocyte alveolar cells.

6d. (B)

6e. (C) Surfactant is indicated for very low birth weight infants as well as larger infants with evidence of pulmonary immaturity. It is prescribed for prophylaxis of infants at high risk of RDS and for treatment of those with RDS.

6f. (A) Exosurf is the only available synthetic surfactant.

6g. (E) The correct dose of Survanta is 4 mL/kg no more than q 6 hours up to 4 doses in the first 48 hours of life. Therefore, Baby Girl Thomas should receive 6 mL per dose (4 mL/kg × 1.5 kg = 6 mL) up to every 6 hours not to exceed 4 doses in the first 48 hours of life.

6h. (D) Pulmonary hemorrhaging is the most concerning adverse effect of surfactant administration and appears to be more common with the synthetic surfactant, Exosurf.

6i. (A) Exosurf is dosed at 5 mL/kg q 12 to 24 hours. It is a lyophilized powder that may be stored at room temperature. During administration, the neonate's head is rotated 45° to each side.

6j. (A)

6k. (C) Survanta is a natural surfactant that contains surfactant-associated proteins B and C and phospholipids 25 mg/mL. The vials are stored under refrigeration and may be swirled gently, but not shaken, if settling occurs.

6l. (D) Maternal steroids may be administered in an attempt to avoid RDS or enhance the neonate's response to surfactant. Betamethasone, 12 mg/day for two doses, has been most commonly used.

6m. (B) Lasix (furosemide) is a loop diuretic that may result in renal elimination of potassium.

CASE 7

7a. (E) Bronchopulmonary dysplasia (BPD) is characterized by oxygen dependence, radiographic abnormalities, and chronic respiratory symptoms persisting for > 28 days of life. Common etiologies include prematurity, immature antioxidant systems, supplemental oxygen, and barotrauma from positive pressure ventilation.

7b. (D) Infants with BPD manifest increased caloric expenditures due in part to increased work of breathing. They also exhibit abnormal pulmonary function and altered gas exchange.

7c. (E) Pathophysiologic mechanisms associated with BPD include pulmonary edema, bronchoconstriction, airway hyperreactivity, airway inflammation, and chronic lung injury and repair.

7d. (B) Loop diuretics, such as furosemide (Lasix), increase the renal excretion of calcium that may lead to nephrocalcinosis.

7e. (C) Furosemide, a loop diuretic, increases the renal excretion of potassium. Albuterol, a β-2 agonist, may lead to decreased serum potassium concentrations due to an intracellular shift of potassium.

7f. (A) Spironolactone is only available in an oral dosage form. A 4 mg/mL suspension may be prepared by dissolving eight 25-mg tablets in 50 mLs of simple syrup of which 0.5 mL would represent Baby Girl Daniels' dose (4 mg/mL = 2 mg/x; x = 0.5 mL).

7g. (A) Hydrochlorothiazide is only available in an oral dosage form.

7h. (A) Baby Girl Daniels is prescribed 2 mg. Therefore, 50 mg/5 mL = 2 mg/x; x = 0.2 mL.

7i. (B) Spironolactone is a potassium-sparing diuretic. Others include triamterene and amiloride.

7j. (C) The serum sodium, potassium, and chloride concentrations are low in Baby Girl Daniels. Although each might be prescribed, the addition of spironolactone, a potassium-sparing diuretic, necessitates careful monitoring of the potassium concentration.

7k. (A) The respective trade and generic names are: Aldactone (spironolactone), Dyazide (combined hydrochlorothiazide and triamterene), Bumex (bumetanide), and Diamox (acetazolamide).

7l. (B) Dexamethasone has been the predominant corticosteroid used in the treatment of BPD. Differing strategies have been used—a 42-day weaning regimen being one of the most common.

7m. (E) Systemic corticosteroids have an array of potential adverse effects including hypertension, hyperglycemia, and hypokalemia, all of which may manifest acutely.

7n. (A) An inappropriate steroid weaning regimen could potentially place the patient with an inadequate amount of "endogenous" cortisol that may manifest as hypotension and hypoglycemia.

7o. (B) Given Baby Girl Daniels' number of bands, it is unlikely that an infection is present. Therefore, a reasonable explanation for the increased white blood cell (WBC) count is the administration of corticosteroids. Corticosteroids result in demargination of WBCs resulting in increased numbers of circulating WBCs.

7p. (A) Thiazide diuretics, such as hydrochlorothiazide (HCTZ), result in increased absorption of calcium and increased excretion of potassium. Spironolactone, a potassium-sparing diuretic, may result in increased serum potassium. Therefore, Baby Girl Daniels might exhibit hypokalemia and/or hypercalcemia from her HCTZ therapy and/or hyperkalemia from her spironolactone therapy.

7q. (B) The injectable form of furosemide may be administered orally. Furosemide, a loop diuretic, primarily acts on the ascending limb of the loop of Henle. The use of loop diuretics may also result in a hypochloremic metabolic alkalosis. Furosemide dilutions should not be refrigerated.

7r. (B) In calculating the amount of dexamethasone needed to prepare 20 mL of the 0.25 mg/mL solution: 0.25 mg/mL × 20 mLs = 5 mg needed. Using a stock solution of 4 mg/mL; 4 mg/mL = 5 mg/x; x = 1.25 mLs.

CASE 8

8a. (B) Physiologic jaundice is noted in ~ 60% of term infants and in over 80% of premature infants. The serum bilirubin reaches maximum values of 6 mg/dL between the 2nd and 4th day and 10–12 mg/dL on the 5th to 7th day in term and premature infants, respectively. Physiologic jaundice causes no harm in healthy full-term infants. Kernicterus, bilirubin encephalopathy, is characterized pathologically by bilirubin staining and necrosis of neurons in the basal ganglia, hippocampal cortex, and subthalamic nuclei of the brain.

8b. (C) Pathologic jaundice may be caused by increased production of bilirubin, deficiency of hepatic uptake, impaired conjugation of bilirubin, or increased enterohepatic circulation of bilirubin.

8c. (D) Heme is degraded by heme oxygenase resulting in the release of iron and the formation of carbon monoxide and biliverdin. Biliverdin is then reduced to bilirubin by biliverdin reductase.

8d. (C) The total bilirubin concentration is the sum of the direct and indirect bilirubin. Therefore, 4 mg/dL (direct) + 17 mg/dL (indirect) = 21 mg/dL.

8e. (C) Albumin can bind bilirubin up to a maximum of 8.2 mg of bilirubin per gram of albumin. Therefore, with an albumin concentration of 3 gm/dL, the maximum serum concentration of albumin bound bilirubin would be 25 mg/dL (3 × 8.2 = ~ 25).

8f. (C) Bilirubin can enter the brain when it is not bound to albumin, unconjugated, or if there is damage to the blood-brain barrier.

8g. (A) Sulfur-based medications, such as Bactrim (combination of sulfamethoxazole and trimethoprim) may displace bilirubin from albumin and thus facilitate its entry into the brain.

8h. (B) Phenobarbital may be beneficial in the treatment of hyperbilirubinemia. It appears to be most effective when administered both to the pregnant mother and the newborn.

8i. (A) The dose of Bactrim should be based on the trimethoprim component.

8j. (A) The active ingredients are as follows: Septra (trimethoprim and sulfamethoxazole), Gantanol (sulfamethoxazole), Zosyn (piperacillin and tazobactam), and Gantrisin (sulfisoxazole).

8k. (D) The daily dose = 30 mg (15 mg twice a day); 80 mg/5 mL = 30 mg/x; x = 1.88 mL.

8l. (D) Benzyl alcohol may cause kernicterus by displacing bilirubin from albumin, thus allowing more bilirubin to pass through the blood-brain barrier. The use of benzyl alcohol in newborns is also associated with respiratory difficulties such as a "gasping syndrome."

CASE 9

9a. (C)

9b. (B) The respective brand and generic names are: Hydrodiuril (hydrochlorothiazide), Diuril (chlorothiazide), Enduron (methyclothiazide), and Dyazide (triamterene and hydrochlorothiazide).

9c. (D) Chlorothiazide is a thiazide diuretic and thus increases the renal clearance of potassium. Also, albuterol therapy results in an intracellular shift of potassium that may result in decreased serum potassium concentrations. Enalaprilat is an angiotensin-converting enzyme inhibitor that decreases aldosterone secretion and thus results in retention of potassium. Thus, administering potassium concurrently with enalaprilat warrants careful monitoring.

9d. (C) Administration of the thiazide diuretics (i.e., chlorothiazide) may result in abnormalities including hyperglycemia, hypokalemia, hyperuricemia, hypercalcemia, and hypomagnesemia.

9e. (B) A reasonable initial regimen of enalaprilat for newborns is 5–10 mcg/kg/dose iv q 8–24 h. Therefore, Baby Girl Prince's dose (20 mcg/3.5 kg = 5.7 mcg/kg) is appropriate; however, the dosing interval should be modified.

9f. (B) Captopril is also an angiotensin-converting enzyme inhibitor. Chlorothiazide is a diuretic, atenolol is a beta blocker, and verapamil is a calcium-channel blocker.

9g. (B) Chlorothiazide is a thiazide diuretic that is typically initially dosed at 10–20 mg/kg q 12 h for newborns. Therefore, Baby Girl Prince should receive 35–70 mg po q 12 h (3.5 kg × 10 mg/kg = 35 mg; 3.5 kg × 20 mg/kg = 70 mg). It is also available in an injectable dosage form.

9h. (C) Enalapril is hydrolyzed in the liver to enalaprilat. Enalaprilat is the parenteral form of enalapril and is available as a 1.25 mg/mL solution. As all angiotensin-converting enzyme inhibitors, it may result in increased serum potassium concentrations and is contraindicated in the presence of bilateral renal artery stenosis.

9i. (D) The administration of chlorothiazide will most likely decrease serum potassium concentrations. However, it is likely to lower the blood pressure by providing an additional mechanism of action (renal) with that of the enalaprilat.

9j. (C) Patients often complain of gastric intolerance to potassium chloride. To improve tolerance, it should be diluted prior to administration. Whenever indicated, potassium chloride should be administered orally. There is a greater risk of cardiovascular complications with intravenous potassium chloride administration.

CASE 10

10a. (A) The greatest risk of intraventricular hemorrhaging (IVH) is within the first 3 days of life in newborns that are < 34-weeks gestation and/or less than 1500 grams. Providing sedation to those at risk may be beneficial by minimizing fluctuating cerebral blood flow.

10b. (C) Clinical detection of IVH is often difficult due to ~ 50% of cases being asymptomatic. In the presence of risk factors, an unexplained fall in the hematocrit or failure of the hematocrit to rise with transfusions may be an indication of the presence of IVH.

10c. (C) Papile's classification for IVH: Grade I = germinal matrix hemorrhaging, Grade II = IVH without ventricular dilatation, Grade III = IVH with ventricular dilatation, Grade IV = IVH with parenchymal extension.

10d. (D) Grade IV is the most severe grade of IVH and has the highest incidence of mental and motor handicaps (~ 50%).

10e. (E) Potential outcomes from IVH include seizures, hydrocephalus, hemorrhagic infarction, neurodevelopmental handicaps, metabolic acidosis, apnea, and increased mortality.

10f. (B) Therapy should be initiated within the first 6 hours of life as ~ 35% of IVH episodes occur within this time period.

10g. (D) Indomethacin has been prescribed for the pre-vention of IVH. Potential beneficial actions include decreased prostaglandins, decreased cerebral blood flow, stabilization of cerebral microvasculature, closure of PDA, and prevention of free radical formation.

10h. (C) Potential benefits of phenobarbital for the prevention of IVH include decreased cerebral blood flow, decreased cerebral metabolic rate, blunting of blood pressure swings, decreased catecholamine release, and decreased enzymatic induction.

10i. (C)

10j. (C) The loading dose is 6mg (5 mg/kg × 1.2 kg = 6 mg). Therefore, using a 65, 130, or 100 mg/mL preparation would result in doses too small for an accurate measurement. Using a 10 mg/mL dilution, 0.6 mL (10 mg/mL = 6 mg/x; x = 0.6) would be the loading dose and could be accurately measured.

10k. (A)

10l. (A) The use of both corticosteroids and aminoglycosides along with neuromuscular blocking agents (i.e., vecuronium) has resulted in increased neuromuscular toxicity (myopathy, prolonged paralysis) and warrants close monitoring in such patients. In this case, the patient is only prescribed an aminoglycoside (gentamicin).

10m. (C)

10n. (E) Prevention is the key in the "treatment" of IVH. Minimizing fluctuations and increases in cerebral blood flow, minimizing acute changes in arterial blood pressure, and minimizing coagulation complications are key.

CASE 11

11a. (D) PPHN is an acronym for persistent pulmonary hypertension that is also referred to as persistent fetal circulation.

11b. (D) PPHN results in blood being shunted away from the lungs resulting in hypoxemia with consequent vasoconstriction. Treatment is directed at promoting pulmonary vasodilation. Hyperventilation, nitric oxide, and extracorporeal membrane oxygenation (ECMO) support are several treatment options.

11c. (B)

11d. (D) ECMO requires the use of heparin to maintain patency of the circuit. The circuit is also known to alter the disposition of select drugs resulting in changes in their pharmacokinetic and pharmacodynamic properties.

11e. (E) Basically, the ECMO circuit uses either a venoarterial or venovenous connection, a reservoir, roller pump, membrane oxygenator, and heat exchanger.

11f. (B) The ECMO circuit (membrane oxygenator) is known to remove certain drugs such as fentanyl. Therefore, excessive doses are often necessary to achieve desired effects in patients receiving ECMO support.

11g. (A) Nitric oxide (NO) is an endothelium-derived relaxing factor that exerts its effects by activation of cyclic GMP. When administered via inhalation, it acts as a pulmonary vasodilator. Nitrous oxide is known as "laughing gas."

11h. (C) Methemoglobinemia results from exposure to chemicals (i.e., nitric oxide) that oxidize the iron in hemoglobin from its ferrous to ferric state. Methemoglobin is unable to carry oxygen and when present in excess results in a functional anemia.

11i. (D) Nitric oxide is dosed in parts per million (PPM).

11j. (B)

11k. (B) ACT is a rapid test that can be performed at the patient's bedside allowing for immediate changes in heparin dosing when indicated.

11l. (D) The correct dopamine dose would be 10 mcg/kg/min. Normal dosing range is from 1–20 mcg/kg/min.

11m.(B) Heparin is dosed in units/kg/hr.

CASE 12

12a. (A) The respective brand and generic names are: Claforan (cefotaxime), Rocephin (ceftriaxone), Fortaz (ceftazidime), and Ceftin (cefuroxime).

12b. (C)

12c. (A) An appropriate dose of cefotaxime for a 38-week gestation newborn is 50 mg/kg iv q 8 h. Therefore, Baby Boy Harris should receive 150 mg iv q 8 h (50 mg/kg × 3 kg = 150 mg).

12d. (E) During most of gestation, a healthy placenta protects the fetus in utero from HIV in maternal blood. However, mixing of the two circulations may occur if the integrity of placental protection is breached via infections or drugs. The majority of transmission occurs around the time of delivery with the remainder occurring late in the third trimester. For breast-feeding women, the risk of transmission is ~ 25–45% with the risk being ~ 15–25% among non–breast-feeding mothers.

12e. (D)

12f. (B)

12g. (D) During labor and delivery, the mother should receive intravenous AZT 2 mg/kg over 1 hour followed by an infusion of 1 mg/kg per hour until clamping of the umbilical cord.

12h. (D) The correct dose of AZT for newborns of HIV infected mothers is 2 mg/kg orally every 6 hours. Therefore, Baby Boy Harris should receive 6 mg po q 6 h (2 mg/kg × 3 kg = 6 mg).

12i. (A)

12j. (B)

MODULE 2

Pediatric Intensive Care

*A truly successful man need not
advertise his accomplishments*

This section consists of 20 medication orders followed by corresponding patient profiles representing pharmacotherapy associated with patients admitted to a pediatric intensive care unit. Each patient profile is followed by multiple-choice questions pertaining to the medication order and profile information. Choose the one best-lettered response to each item. The correct answers are provided at the end of this section. The reader is encouraged to attempt all questions for each case or for the entire section prior to referring to the answer key. Moreover, where appropriate, the answer key provides a thorough explanation of the correct response and should serve as an additional learning tool for the reader.

CASE 1

PHYSICIAN ORDER

Patient Weight: <u>45 kg</u>

Ipratropium bromide 500 mcg inh q 6 h
Fluticasone inhaler 2 puffs bid

Date/Time: <u>07/21/0900</u>
Physician: <u>John Wright</u>

Patient Name: <u>Carlos Smith</u>
Patient ID #: <u>213430</u>

MEDICAL PROFILE

Patient: Carlos Smith

Patient Weight: 45 kg   **Age:** 11 y/o

Present Illness: Status asthmaticus

Allergies: None

Medical History: Asthma, "cold" over the past few days

Labs: Na 136, K 4.2, Cl 107, C02 21, Cr 0.6, BUN 7, Glu 115, Ca 9.1, Lactate 1.1, WBC 5000, H/H 12.2/36.6, Plat 260,000, Segs 86%, Bands 4%

ABG: pH 7.47, PCO_2 30, PO_2 50, HCO_3 23

Cultures: Pending

Medication Profile:

Date	Medication
7/21/0800	Albuterol 2.5 mg neb q 5 minutes × 3, then q 1 h

1a.   Asthma is characterized by airway

_____.

A.   inflammation
B.   hyperresponsiveness
C.   obstruction
D.   A and B only
E.   A, B, and C

1b.   Which of the following is recognized as the central component of the pathophysiology of asthma?

A.   Inflammation
B.   Hyperresponsiveness
C.   Obstruction
D.   Bronchoconstriction

1c.   Which of the following is associated with the pathophysiology of asthma?

A.   Macrophages
B.   Mast cells
C.   Eosinophils
D.   B and C only
E.   A, B, and C

1d.   Which of the following is a cardinal symptom suggestive of asthma?

A.   Wheezing
B.   Breathlessness
C.   Coughing
D.   A and B only
E.   A, B, and C

1e. Which of the following is a brand name for albuterol?

A. Ventolin
B. Vancenase
C. Flovent
D. Vanceril

1f. Which of the following lab values would most likely be altered by the administration of albuterol?

A. Chloride
B. Potassium
C. Sodium
D. Calcium

1g. Which of the following would be a more appropriate albuterol regimen for Carlos?

A. 2.5 mg neb q 1 minute × 3, then q 1 h
B. 2.5 mg neb q 20 minutes × 3, then q 1 h
C. 2.5 mg neb q 1 h × 3, then q 2 h
D. The albuterol regimen is correct as prescribed

1h. Which of the following is a brand name for ipratropium bromide?

A. Proventil
B. Serevent
C. Atrovent
D. Flovent

1i. Ipratropium bromide is classified as a(n) _____.

A. β-2 agonist
B. β-1 agonist
C. β-2 antagonist
D. anticholinergic

1j. The name brand for fluticasone is _____.

A. Vancenase
B. Flovent
C. Serevent
D. Azmacort

1k. Fluticasone is classified as a(n) _____.

A. β-2 agonist
B. corticosteroid
C. anticholinergic
D. mast cell stabilizer

1l. Which of the following is true regarding the fluticasone order for Carlos?

A. Is correct as prescribed
B. Should be changed to 2 puffs qid
C. Should be discontinued and substituted with systemic methylprednisolone
D. Should be changed to 1 mg/kg iv bid

CASE 2

PHYSICIAN ORDER

Patient Weight: 55 lbs

Aminophylline 1 mg/kg loading dose followed by 0.5 mg/kg/hr
Obtain aminophylline concentrations per protocol

Date/Time: 08/22/0900
Physician: Sam Thompkins

Patient Name: Ali Levin
Patient ID #: 213145

MEDICAL PROFILE

Patient: Ali Levin

Patient Weight: 55 lbs   **Age:** 6 y/o

Present Illness: Status asthmaticus, febrile

Allergies: None

Medical History: Asthma

Labs: Na 137, K 3.9, Cl 108, C02 22, Cr 0.5, BUN 4, Glu 130, Ca 9.1, Lactate 1.4, WBC 14000, H/H 11.9/36, Plat 350,000, Segs 74%, Bands 24%, Lymphs 2%, Monos 0%, CRP 4

ABG: pH 7.40, PCO_2 40, PO_2 70, HCO_3 24

Cultures: Pending

Medication Profile:

Date	Medication
8/21/0900	Albuterol 2.5 mg neb q 2 h
8/21/0900	Ipratropium bromide 500 mcg neb q 4 h
8/21/0900	Methylprednisolone 2.5 mg iv q 6 h
8/21/0900	Azithromycin 25 mg iv qd

2a. The drug of choice for the initial treatment of status asthmaticus is a(n) _____.

    A. corticosteroid
    B. β-2 agonist
    C. anticholinergic
    D. leukotriene antagonist

2b. Which of the following is a brand name of methylprednisolone?

    A. Solu-Cortef
    B. Celestone
    C. Pediapred
    D. Solu-Medrol

2c. Methylprednisolone is classified as a(n) _____.

    A. β-2 agonist
    B. corticosteroid
    C. anticholinergic
    D. methylxanthine

2d. Which of the following is true regarding the methylprednisolone prescribed for Ali?

    A. Is correct as prescribed
    B. Correct dose is 25 mg iv q 6 h
    C. Dose is correct, but should only be prescribed every 12 hours
    D. Should be discontinued prior to initiating aminophylline therapy
    E. Both B and D are correct

2e. Methylprednisolone is available as a 20 mg/mL solution for injection. How many milliliters of this stock solution are needed for each dose as prescribed to Ali?

    A. 0.5 mL
    B. 0.13 mL
    C. 8 mL
    D. 2 mL

2f. Which of the following is a potential adverse effect from methylprednisolone therapy?

    I. Hypoglycemia
    II. Hypertension
    III. Adrenal suppression

        A. I only
        B. III only
        C. I and III
        D. II and III
        E. I, II, and III

2g. Which of the following drugs is most similar to azithromycin?

    A. Ciprofloxacin
    B. Clarithromycin
    C. Aztreonam
    D. Ticarcillin

2h. Which of the following is true regarding Ali's azithromycin therapy?

    A. It will likely result in increased theophylline serum concentrations
    B. It will likely result in decreased theophylline serum concentrations
    C. It will likely not affect theophylline serum concentrations
    D. Theophylline therapy will likely alter the activity of azithromycin

2i. The appropriate dose of azithromycin for Ali is _____.

    A. As prescribed
    B. 125 mg iv q 12 h
    C. 250 mg iv qd
    D. 10 mg/kg iv × 1, then 5 mg/kg iv qd

2j. Azithromycin was most likely prescribed for Ali because of its activity against _____.

    A. *Pseudomonas*
    B. *Staphylococcus aureus*
    C. *Staphylococcus epidermidis*
    D. *Mycoplasma*

2k. Aminophylline is classified as a(n) _____.

    A. β-2 agonist
    B. leukotriene antagonist
    C. methylxanthine
    D. anticholinergic

2l. Which of the following is a brand name for aminophylline?

    A. Somophyllin
    B. Elixophyllin
    C. Slo-bid
    D. Theo-dur

2m. A more appropriate aminophylline loading dose for Ali would be _____ milligrams.

    A. 50
    B. 100
    C. 150
    D. 200

2n. A more appropriate aminophylline maintenance dose for Ali would be _____ mg/hr.

    A. 12
    B. 18
    C. 25
    D. 50

2o. Which of the following is a reasonable targeted therapeutic serum concentration of theophylline?

    A. 5–10 mcg/mL
    B. 5–15 mg/L
    C. 20–30 mcg/mL
    D. 20–40 mg/L

2p. Which of the following is the rationale for prescribing an aminophylline-loading dose to Ali?

   A. Allows for rapid achievement of steady-state concentrations
   B. Results in potentially less adverse effects
   C. Allows for rapid achievement of a desired concentration
   D. Allows the nurse to administer the first dose while pharmacy prepares the maintenance infusion

CASE 3

PHYSICIAN ORDER

Patient Weight: <u>60 kg</u>

Magnesium sulfate 25 mg/kg iv loading dose followed by 20 mg/kg/min
Obtain magnesium concentration postbolus dose.

Date/Time: <u>09/22/1000</u>   **Patient Name:** <u>Andre Green</u>
Physician: <u>Ellen Troy</u>   **Patient ID #:** <u>212545</u>

MEDICAL PROFILE

Patient: Andre Green   **Patient Weight:** 60 kg   **Age:** 12 y/o

Present Illness: Refractory status asthmaticus,   **Allergies:** None
intubated, and on mechanical ventilator

Medical History: Asthma, multiple ICU admissions

Labs: Na 140, K 4, Cl 110, C02 23, Cr 0.5, BUN 8, Glu 150, Ca 8.1, Mg 2.1, Lactate 2, WBC 16000,
H/H 13/39.6, Plat 390,000, Segs 80%, Bands 4%, Lymphs 6%, Monos 5%, CRP 0.5, Theophylline 13

ABG: pH 7.33, PCO_2 55, PO_2 65, HCO_3 24

Cultures: Pending

Medication Profile:

Date	Medication
9/21/1600	Albuterol 2.5 mg neb q 1 h
9/21/1600	Ipratropium bromide 500 mcg neb q 2 h
9/21/1600	Methylprednisolone 60 mg iv q 6 h
9/21/2300	Aminophylline 0.7 mg/kg/hr
9/21/2300	Fentanyl 60 mcg/hr
9/21/2300	Vecuronium 0.1 mg/kg/hr
9/21/2300	Ranitidine 1 mg/kg iv q 12 h

3a. Which of the following is a proposed mechanism of action of magnesium in the treatment of asthma?

A. Induces the degranulation of mast cells
B. Increases the concentration of acetylcholine at motor nerve terminals
C. Antagonizes the translocation of calcium across cell membranes
D. A and B only
E. A, B, and C

3b. Which of the following is a sign of magnesium toxicity?

A. Hypotension
B. Muscle weakness
C. Respiratory depression
D. A and B only
E. A, B, and C

3c. A reasonable targeted serum magnesium concentration in Andre would be _____ mg/dL.

    A. 1.6–2.2
    B. 4–5
    C. 5–7
    D. 7–9

3d. Which of the following would be a more appropriate magnesium regimen for Andre?

    A. 2 gram-loading dose, then 20 mg/kg/min
    B. 2 gram-loading dose, then 20 mg/kg/hr
    C. 25 mg/kg loading dose, then 50 mg/kg/min
    D. 25 mg/kg loading dose, then 2 gm/hr

3e. Magnesium sulfate is available as an 80 mg/2 mL solution for injection. How many milliliters are needed to prepare the prescribed loading dose for Andre?

    A. 0.625 mL
    B. 1.25 mL
    C. 18.75 mL
    D. 37.5 mL

3f. An intravenous solution is prepared for Andre that contains aminophylline 500 mg/500 mL. At what rate should this preparation be infused to provide Andre with his prescribed dose?

    A. 12 mL/hr
    B. 42 mL/hr
    C. 60 mL/min
    D. 70 mL/min

3g. Which of the following medications is prescribed incorrectly for Andre?

    A. Albuterol
    B. Methylprednisolone
    C. Vecuronium
    D. Ranitidine

3h. What is the most likely reason for prescribing ranitidine to Andre?

    A. Treatment of peptic ulcer disease
    B. Treatment of gastroesophageal reflux
    C. Prophylaxis for stress ulcers
    D. Prophylaxis for nausea and vomiting

3i. Which of the following medications most closely resembles ranitidine?

    A. Famotidine
    B. Metoclopramide
    C. Omeprazole
    D. Magnesium hydroxide

3j. Which of the following medications may have likely been substituted for ranitidine?

    A. Omeprazole
    B. Metoclopramide
    C. Ondansetron
    D. Bismuth salicylate

CASE 4

PHYSICIAN ORDER

Patient Weight: <u>40 kg</u>

Ketamine 0.5 mg/kg loading dose followed by 1 mg/kg/min

Date/Time: <u>11/21/1000</u>   **Patient Name:** <u>David Michaels</u>
Physician: <u>Brad Moser</u>   **Patient ID #:** <u>782545</u>

MEDICAL PROFILE

Patient: David Michaels   **Patient Weight:** 40 kg   **Age:** 16 y/o

Present Illness: Respiratory distress, mechanical ventilation   **Allergies:** Peanuts

Medical History: Asthma, multiple hospital and ICU admissions

Labs: Na 138, K 3.7, Cl 107, C02 18, Cr 0.7, BUN 10, Glu 180, Ca 7.9, Mg 4.1, Lactate 5.1, WBC 7000, H/H 13/38, Plat 225,000, Segs 84%, Bands 12%, Lymphs 4%, Monos 2%, CRP 0.3, theophylline 12

ABG: pH 7.30, PCO_2 50, PO_2 60, HCO_3 22

Cultures: Pending

Medication Profile:

Date	Medication
11/19/1500	Albuterol 2.5 mg neb q 2 h
11/19/1500	Ipratropium bromide 500 mcg neb q 4 h
11/19/1500	Methylprednisolone 40 mg iv q 6 h
11/19/1500	Azithromycin 400 mg iv q 12 h
11/19/2300	Aminophylline 30 mg/hr
11/20/1000	Lorazepam 0.01 mg/kg/min
11/20/1000	Vecuronium 0.15 mg/kg/hr
11/20/1000	Ranitidine 40 mg iv
11/20/2000	Magnesium sulfate 800 mg/hr

4a. Which of the following would be a more appropriate ketamine regimen for David?

   A. 0.5 mg/kg loading dose followed by 40 mg/hr
   B. 0.5 mg/kg loading dose followed by 1 mcg/kg/min
   C. 1 mg/kg loading dose followed by 0.1 mg/kg/min
   D. 1 mg/kg loading dose followed by 1 mg/kg/min

4b. Which of the following is the proposed mechanism of action of ketamine for the treatment of asthma?

   A. Increases synaptic catecholamine concentrations
   B. Inhibits degranulation of mast cells
   C. Leukotriene inhibition
   D. Increases acetylcholine activity on bronchial smooth muscles

4c. Which of the following is a potential adverse effect of ketamine therapy?

   A. Increased oral and tracheal secretions
   B. Cardiovascular stimulation
   C. Increased intraocular pressure
   D. A and B only
   E. A, B, and C

4d. Which of the following might be prescribed to David in an attempt to counteract the side effects of ketamine therapy?

   A. Atropine
   B. Fentanyl
   C. Dopamine
   D. Diazepam

4e. Which of the following is the brand name of azithromycin?

   A. Biaxin
   B. Zithromax
   C. Azactam
   D. E-mycin

4f. Which of the following is true regarding the azithromycin prescribed for David?

   A. It should be substituted with clarithromycin
   B. It should be substituted with erythromycin
   C. The dose should be adjusted
   D. It should only be administered orally

4g. Lorazepam is classified as a(n) _____.

   A. opiate
   B. antidepressant
   C. neuromuscular blocking agent
   D. benzodiazepine

4h. Which of the following is an appropriate dose of lorazepam for David?

   A. 0.01 mcg/kg/min
   B. 0.01 mg/kg/min
   C. 0.1 mg/kg/min
   D. 0.1 mg/kg/hr

4i. How many milligrams of vecuronium will David receive per day?

   A. 6 mg
   B. 12 mg
   C. 72 mg
   D. 144 mg

4j. Given the potential for enhanced adverse effects, the coadministration of vecuronium and _____ necessitates increased patient monitoring.

   A. lorazepam
   B. methylprednisolone
   C. aminophylline
   D. ranitidine

4k. The ranitidine prescribed for David should be administered every ____ hours.

   A. 4
   B. 8
   C. 12
   D. 24

4l. Ranitidine for injection is supplied as a 25 mg/mL solution. How many milliliters are needed to provide each prescribed dose for David?

   A. 0.63 mL
   B. 1.25 mL
   C. 1.6 mL
   D. 3.2 mL

4m. Given the reported magnesium concentration in David, the magnesium infusion should be _____.

A. discontinued for 1 hour and then restarted at 10 mg/kg/hr
B. discontinued for 2 hours and then restarted at 10 mg/kg/hr
C. decreased to 10 mg/kg/hr
D. maintained as prescribed

4n. Which of David's reported lab values may have been affected by albuterol therapy?

A. Sodium
B. Chloride
C. Lactate
D. Platelets

4o. If David was initially given a 6 mg/kg loading dose of aminophylline, what would have been the theophylline peak concentration obtained after the loading dose? (volume of distribution = 0.5 L/kg, elimination rate constant = 0.174/hr)

A. 3.4 mg/L
B. 8.2 mg/L
C. 9.6 mg/L
D. 12.5 mg/L

CASE 5

PHYSICIAN ORDER

Patient Weight: <u>40 kg</u>

Fosphenytoin 10 mg/kg PE iv loading dose over 60 minutes followed by 5 mg/kg/day divided every 12 hours. Obtain phenytoin peak concentration after the loading dose.

Date/Time: <u>10/16/1000</u>
Physician: <u>John Stephens</u>

Patient Name: <u>Donte Richards</u>
Patient ID #: <u>782545</u>

MEDICAL PROFILE

Patient: Donte Richards

Patient Weight: 40 kg   **Age:** 12 y/o

Present Illness: Motor vehicle accident, status epilepticus, seizure terminated with second dose of lorazepam in emergency department

Allergies: PCN

Medical History: Unremarkable

Labs: Na 140, K 4.3, Cl 112, C02 23.5, Cr 0.8, BUN 7, Glu 117, Ca 8.2, Mg 1.8, WBC 14000, H/H 11.9/34.8, Plat 178,000, Segs 42%, Bands 53%, Lymphs 3%, Monos 1%, CRP 11.3, Alb 3.5

Cultures: Pending

Medication Profile:

Date	Medication
10/16/0900	Lorazepam 0.01 mg/kg prn seizure activity
10/16/0900	Oxacillin 2 gms iv q 6 h
10/16/0900	Ranitidine 40 mg iv q 8 h
10/16/0900	Morphine sulfate 4 mg iv q 2 h prn pain

5a. Which of the following is true regarding status epilepticus?

   A. Defined as continuous seizure activity for longer than 60 minutes
   B. Is one of the most common life-threatening emergencies among children
   C. Defined as the occurrence of two or more seizures without full recovery of consciousness during the interictal period
   D. B and C only
   E. A, B, and C

5b. Which of the following is a potential etiology of status epilepticus?

   A. Head trauma
   B. Infections
   C. Tumors
   D. A and B only
   E. A, B, and C

5c. During the early stages of status epilepticus, manifestations of increased autonomic discharge include _____.

    A. bradycardia
    B. hypotension
    C. hypoglycemia
    D. hyperthermia

5d. Which of the following is the drug of choice for the initial treatment of status epilepticus?

    A. Phenytoin
    B. Phenobarbital
    C. Lorazepam
    D. Diazepam

5e. Which of the following is true of lorazepam compared with diazepam in the treatment of status epilepticus?

    A. Is less lipid soluble
    B. Faster onset of action
    C. Longer duration of action
    D. A and C only
    E. A, B, and C

5f. Which of the following is true regarding fosphenytoin?

    A. Is less water soluble than phenytoin
    B. May only be administered intravenously
    C. Does not contain propylene glycol
    D. Both B and C

5g. Which of the following is true regarding the fosphenytoin-loading dose for Donte?

    A. Is correct as prescribed
    B. Should be changed to 20 mg/kg PE and infused at a faster rate
    C. Should be changed to 20 mg/kg PE and infused at a slower rate
    D. Correct dose is prescribed, but should be infused at a faster rate

5h. What does the term "PE" signify in the fosphenytoin order?

    A. Phenytoin sodium equivalents
    B. Phenytoin equal
    C. Phenytoin extract
    D. Phenytoin sodium extract

5i. At what time should the requested phenytoin concentration be obtained?

    A. Immediately after the loading dose is infused
    B. 1 hour postinfusion
    C. 2 hours postinfusion
    D. 6 hours postinfusion

5j. What is the equivalent phenytoin dose to the fosphenytoin dose prescribed to Donte?

    A. 6.7 mg/kg
    B. 10 mg/kg
    C. 15 mg/kg
    D. 20 mg/kg

5k. In the treatment of status epilepticus, an initial desired peak concentration of phenytoin would be _____.

    A. 5–10 mcg/mL
    B. 10–15 mcg/mL
    C. 15–20 mg/L
    D. 20–30 mg/L

5l. The brand name for fosphenytoin is _____.

    A. Celebrex
    B. Cerebyx
    C. Cefadyl
    D. Cedax

5m. Which of Donte's medications is prescribed incorrectly?

    A. Lorazepam
    B. Oxacillin
    C. Ranitidine
    D. Morphine

5n. What is the maximum recommended single dose of lorazepam for Donte?

    A. 1 mg
    B. 2 mg
    C. 3 mg
    D. 4 mg

CASE 6

PHYSICIAN ORDER

Patient Weight: 27 kg

Midazolam 1 mg/kg iv loading dose, then 10 mcg/kg/min
Titrate as needed for resolution of seizure

Date/Time: 2/28/1000   **Patient Name:** Jenny Spiller
Physician: Chris Roberts   **Patient ID #:** 784785

MEDICAL PROFILE

Patient: Jenny Spiller   **Patient Weight:** 27 kg   **Age:** 6 y/o

Present Illness: Status epilepticus, intubated,   **Allergies:** None
on mechanical ventilator

Medical History: Partial Seizures

Labs: Na 140, K 4, Cl 102, C02 26.1, Cr 0.4, BUN 10, Glu 85, Ca 8, Mg 2.1, WBC 10800, H/H 10.3/33, Plat 450,000, Segs 65%, Bands 12%, Lymphs 13%, Monos 10%, Alb 3.8, phenytoin 9

Medication Profile:

Date	Medication
2/28/0200	Lorazepam 0.1 mg/kg prn seizure activity
2/28/0300	Phenytoin 1 mg/kg iv q 12 h
2/28/0300	Ranitidine 30 mg iv q 8 h
2/28/0400	Phenobarbital 2.5 mg/kg iv q 12 h
2/28/0400	Fentanyl 27 mcg/hr

6a. The maximum recommended rate of infusion of the phenytoin prescribed for Jenny is _____.

   A. 1 mg/kg/min
   B. 3 mg/kg/min
   C. 10 mg/hr
   D. 30 mg/hr

6b. Which of the following is true regarding Jenny's phenytoin regimen?

   A. Is correct as prescribed
   B. Initial maintenance regimen should be 1 mg/kg iv q 8 h
   C. Initial maintenance regimen should be 2.5 mg/kg iv q 12 h
   D. Initial maintenance regimen should be 2.5 mg/kg iv q 8 h

6c. Based on Jenny's reported phenytoin concentration, the most appropriate action would be to _____.

   A. hold the next dose and resume at 30 mg iv qd
   B. bolus with 5 mg/kg and increase maintenance dose to 70 mg iv q 12 h
   C. bolus with 10 mg/kg and maintain same maintenance dose
   D. bolus with 10 mg/kg and increase maintenance dose to 70 mg iv q 12 h

6d. A phenytoin bolus dose of 200 mg would increase Jenny's phenytoin concentration to approximately _____ mg/L. (phenytoin's volume of distribution = 0.7 L/kg, half-life = 10 hours)

   A. 15
   B. 20
   C. 25
   D. 30

6e. Phenobarbital is classified as a _____.

   A. sedative
   B. benzodiazepine
   C. barbiturate
   D. hydantoin

6f. Which of the following is true regarding Jenny's phenobarbital therapy?

   A. Should be modified to 2.5 mg/kg iv qd
   B. Should be modified to 2.5 mg/kg iv q 8 h
   C. Should be discontinued prior to initiating midazolam therapy
   D. Is appropriate as prescribed

6g. An appropriate initial phenobarbital-loading dose for Jenny would have been _____ milligrams.

   A. 30
   B. 150
   C. 300
   D. 550

6h. The recommended therapeutic serum concentration of phenobarbital is _____.

   A. 5–10 mcg/mL
   B. 10–20 mcg/mL
   C. 15–40 mcg/mL
   D. 40–50 mcg/mL

6i. Which of the following is true of midazolam?

   A. Is a water-soluble benzodiazepine
   B. Has proven efficacy in the treatment of refractory status epilepticus
   C. Has the longest half-life among the parental benzodiazepines
   D. A and B only
   E. A, B, and C

6j. A more appropriate initial midazolam regimen for Jenny would be _____.

   A. 1 mg/kg loading dose, then 1 mcg/kg/min
   B. 1 mg/kg loading dose, then 1 mcg/kg/hr
   C. 0.15 mg/kg loading dose, then 10 mcg/kg/min
   D. 0.15 mg/kg loading dose, then 1 mcg/kg/min

6k. A brand name of midazolam is _____.

   A. Valium
   B. Versed
   C. Vasotec
   D. Ventolin

6l. Which of the following medications most resembles midazolam?

   A. Diprivan
   B. Dilantin
   C. Diazepam
   D. Demadex

6m. Which of the following is a potential adverse effect of midazolam therapy?

   A. Apnea
   B. Hypotension
   C. Sedation
   D. A and C only
   E. A, B, and C

6n. Once Jenny's seizure activity is controlled, what would be the most appropriate strategy to discontinue her midazolam therapy?

   A. Discontinue infusion and administer bolus doses as needed
   B. Wean infusion by 1–2 mcg/kg/min every 15 minutes until discontinued
   C. Switch to oral midazolam and wean by 10% every 2 hours
   D. Discontinue and administer lorazepam bolus doses as prescribed

CASE 7

PHYSICIAN ORDER

Patient Weight: 35 kg

Discontinue pentobarbital
Propofol 3 mg/kg/hr

Date/Time: 3/14/2300
Physician: Steve Ulrich

Patient Name: Sam Smyth
Patient ID #: 745545

MEDICAL PROFILE

Patient: Sam Smyth

Patient Weight: 35 kg   **Age:** 10 y/o

Present Illness: Refractory status epilepticus, mechanical ventilation

Allergies: None

Medical History: Complex partial seizures

Labs: Na 139, K 4.7, Cl 103, C02 26.2, Cr 0.6, BUN 8, Glu 95, Ca 8, Mg 2.1, Alb 4, phenytoin 17, pentobarbital pending

Medication Profile:

Date	Medication
3/14/1500	Lorazepam 4 mg iv prn
3/14/1500	Phenytoin 90 mg iv q 12 h
3/14/1500	Ranitidine 40 mg iv q 8 h
3/14/1800	Fentanyl 35 mcg/hr
3/14/1900	Pentobarbital 70 mg/hr

7a. Pentobarbital is classified as a(n) _____.

  A. benzodiazepine
  B. barbiturate
  C. opiate
  D. phenol

7b. An appropriate loading dose of pentobarbital for Sam would have been _____.

  A. 350 mg infused over 5–10 minutes
  B. 350 mg infused over 1–2 hours
  C. 700 mg infused over 5–10 minutes
  D. 700 mg infused over 30 minutes

7c. A reasonable targeted serum concentration of pentobarbital for Sam would be _____ mg/L.

  A. 1–5
  B. 5–10
  C. 10–20
  D. 20–40

7d. Pentobarbital is supplied as a 50 mg/mL solution. How many milliliters are needed to provide Sam's daily dose as prescribed?

  A. 16 mL
  B. 34 mL
  C. 63 mL
  D. 70 mL

7e. The brand name of pentobarbital is

_____.

A. Seconal
B. Nembutal
C. Mebaral
D. Solfoton

7f. The brand name of propofol is

_____.

A. Ditropan
B. Diprivan
C. Demadex
D. Dalmane

7g. Propofol (10 mg/mL) is supplied in a 10% intralipid emulsion. How many grams of intralipids will Sam receive per day?

A. 10 gms
B. 25 gms
C. 100 gms
D. 250 gms

7h. Which laboratory value should be routinely monitored during propofol therapy?

A. Sodium
B. Magnesium
C. Triglycerides
D. Albumin

7i. Which of the following is true of propofol?

A. Sedative effects usually dissipate within 15–30 minutes of discontinuation
B. Potential adverse effects include hypotension and apnea
C. During administration, intravenous tubing should be replaced every 12 hours
D. A and B only
E. A, B, and C

7j. Besides resolution of seizure activity, an additional potential advantage of propofol therapy for Sam is

_____.

A. induction of phenytoin metabolism
B. inhibition of lorazepam clearance
C. decrease in intracranial pressure
D. decrease in amino acid requirements

7k. What is the maximum recommended infusion rate for the phenytoin dose prescribed for Sam?

A. 35 mg/min
B. 50 mg/min
C. 70 mg/min
D. 90 mg/min

7l. Phenytoin is supplied as a 50 mg/mL solution for injection. How many milliliters are required to provide Sam with his daily dose?

A. 1.8 mL
B. 3.6 mL
C. 5.4 mL
D. 7.2 mL

CASE 8

PHYSICIAN ORDER

Patient Weight: 40 kg

Pentobarbital 1 mg/kg loading dose followed by 1 mg/kg/hr

Date/Time: 1/14/2300
Physician: Noah White

Patient Name: Cary Pender
Patient ID #: 635545

MEDICAL PROFILE

Patient: Cary Pender

Patient Weight: 40 kg   **Age:** 11 y/o

Present Illness: Head trauma, elevated ICP (22 mmHg), mechanical ventilation

Medical History: Previously healthy

Labs: Na 135, K 3.8, Cl 107, C02 21, Cr 0.6, BUN 7, Glu 150, Ca 8.3, Mg 2, WBC 14000, H/H 12/37, Plat 250,000, Segs 42%, Bands 23%, Lymphs 2%, Monos 3%, CRP 9.3

Vitals: B/P 120/60, R 22, P 90, T 38.5 C

Cultures: Pending

Medication Profile:

Date	Medication
1/14/0600	Mannitol 100 mg/kg iv q 12 h
1/14/0600	Oxacillin 2 gms iv q 6 h
1/14/0600	Ranitidine 40 mg iv q 8 h
1/14/0600	Fentanyl 40 mcg/hr
1/14/2300	Vecuronium 0.1 mg/kg/hr

8a. Which of the following is associated with increased intracranial pressure?

    A. Hypertension
    B. Fixed pupils
    C. Bradycardia
    D. A and B only
    E. A, B, and C

8b. An intracranial pressure value exceeding _____ mm Hg is considered abnormal.

    A. 5
    B. 10
    C. 12
    D. 15

8c. What is the calculated cerebral perfusion pressure for Cary?

A. 50 mm Hg
B. 58 mm Hg
C. 60 mm Hg
D. 68 mm Hg

8d. Cerebral blood flow virtually ceases when cerebral perfusion pressure falls below _____ mm Hg.

A. 20
B. 30
C. 40
D. 50

8e. Which of the following are devices used to continuously monitor intracranial pressure?

A. Epidural catheter
B. Intraventricular catheter
C. Subarachnoid bolt
D. A and B only
E. A, B, and C

8f. Mannitol is classified as a(n) _____.

A. carbonic anhydrase inhibitor
B. osmotic diuretic
C. loop diuretic
D. potassium-sparing diuretic

8g. Which of the following laboratory values should be routinely monitored in patients receiving mannitol therapy?

A. osmolality
B. glucose
C. mannitol serum concentrations
D. chloride

8h. What is the calculated serum osmolality in Cary?

A. 250 mOsm/L
B. 281 mOsm/L
C. 295 mOsm/L
D. 315 mOsm/L

8i. A decision to **withhold mannitol dosing** would most likely occur if Cary's serum osmolality exceeded _____ mOsm/L.

A. 280
B. 300
C. 310
D. 320

8j. The duration of action of mannitol is approximately _____ hours.

A. 2
B. 4
C. 6
D. 8

8k. Which of the following is a more appropriate mannitol regimen for Cary?

A. 4000 mg iv q 8 hours
B. 4 grams iv q 4 hours
C. 10,000 mg iv q 8 hours
D. 10 grams iv q 4 hours

8l. Besides mannitol, what other therapy might be prescribed to lower Cary's intracranial pressure?

A. Propofol
B. 3% saline
C. 23.4% saline
D. A and B only
E. A, B, and C

8m. Which of the following is true regarding hyperventilation as a method to lower intracranial pressure?

A. Results in a decrease in the arterial carbon dioxide tension
B. Decreased PCO_2 results in cerebral vasodilatation leading to reduced cerebral blood volume
C. When hyperventilation is discontinued, the PCO_2 should be allowed to return slowly to normal to prevent rebound elevation of ICP
D. A and C only
E. A, B, and C

8n. Which of the following would be a more appropriate pentobarbital regimen for Cary?

A. 40-mg loading dose, then 5 mg/kg/hr
B. 200-mg loading dose, then 5 mg/kg/hr
C. 400-mg loading dose, then 1 mg/kg/hr
D. 400-mg loading dose, then 5 mg/kg/hr

8o. Which of the following is a potential mechanism of action for pentobarbital in the treatment of increased intracranial pressure?

A. Increases cerebrovascular resistance, thereby lowering cerebral blood flow and volume
B. Increases energy requirements of the brain, thereby maintaining cerebral function
C. Vasodilatation of cerebral vessels resulting in blood being shunted from normal to ischemic areas
D. Vasodilatation of cerebral vessels reducing fluid formation

CASE 9

PHYSICIAN ORDER

Patient Weight: <u>63 kg</u>

Mucomyst 50 mg/kg po q 6 h x 17 doses
Ranitidine 50 mg iv q 8 h
Ondansetron 4 mg iv q 8 h prn

Date/Time: <u>9/14/1400</u>
Physician: <u>Robert Kelly</u>

Patient Name: <u>Melissa Haywood</u>
Patient ID #: <u>745587</u>

MEDICAL PROFILE

Patient: Melissa Haywood   **Patient Weight:** 63 kg   **Age:** 15 y/o

Present Illness: Acetaminophen overdose; ~ 50 extra strength capsules

Medical History: Previously healthy

Labs: Na 137, K 4.1, Cl 99, C02 21, Cr 0.7, BUN 9, Glu 131, acetaminophen 72.1 (12 hours postingestion)

Vitals: B/P 146/88, R 16, P 68

Medication Profile:

9a. Which of the following is a trade name for acetaminophen?

    A. Tylenol
    B. Tempra
    C. Neopap
    D. A and B only
    E. A, B, and C

9b. Which of the following products contain acetaminophen?

    A. Sudafed Severe Cold Formula
    B. Vicks NyQuil
    C. Alka-Seltzer Plus Cold and Cough Tablets
    D. A and B only
    E. A, B, and C

9c. Which of the following is the most concerning adverse effect resulting from an overdose of acetaminophen?

    A. Kidney failure
    B. Hepatic failure
    C. Cor pulmonale (right heart failure)
    D. Gastrointestinal bleeding

9d. The metabolite believed to be responsible for the major toxicity from an acetaminophen overdose is

    _____.

    A. Mercapturic acid
    B. Hydroxyacetaminophen
    C. 6-hydroxyacetaminophen
    D. N-acetylimidoquinone

9e. What other laboratory value might be considered for Melissa to further evaluate potential toxicity induced by her ingestion?

   A. Prothrombin time
   B. GGT
   C. AST
   D. A and C only
   E. A, B, and C

9f. Which of the following laboratory values exhibits the most acute change subsequent to an acetaminophen overdose?

   A. Prothrombin time (PT)
   B. Partial thromboplastin time (PTT)
   C. ALT
   D. AST

9g. The first acetaminophen serum concentration should be obtained no sooner than _____ hours postingestion.

   A. 2
   B. 4
   C. 6
   D. 8

9h. By history, what quantity of acetaminophen was ingested by Melissa?

   A. 150 mg/kg
   B. 300 mg/kg
   C. 400 mg/kg
   D. 500 mg/kg

9i. The active component of Mucomyst is _____.

   A. homocysteine
   B. acetylcysteine
   C. acetylcholine
   D. bromocysteine

9j. Mucomyst is available as a 20% solution. How many milliliters are needed to provide a single prescribed dose to Melissa?

   A. 1.57 mL
   B. 5.75 mL
   C. 15.75 mL
   D. 157 mL

9k. Prior to receiving her maintenance doses of Mucomyst, a loading dose of _____ should have been administered.

   A. 100 mg/kg
   B. 125 mg/kg
   C. 8,800 mg
   D. 12,600 mg

9l. The rationale for prescribing Mucomyst for acetaminophen overdoses is to _____.

   A. increase the clearance of acetaminophen
   B. bind the acetaminophen and allow for enhanced renal elimination
   C. provide a glutathione substitute
   D. repair damaged tissue resulting from acetaminophen

9m. The _____ Nomogram is used to plot acetaminophen concentrations subsequent to an ingestion to determine the degree of potential toxicity.

   A. Done
   B. Rumack
   C. Nelson
   D. Ross

9n. A more appropriate maintenance dose of Mucomyst for Melissa would be _____.

   A. 50 mg/kg po q 4 h for 17 doses
   B. 70 mg/kg po q 4 h for 17 doses
   C. 70 mg/kg po q 6 h for 17 doses
   D. 50 mg/kg po × 4 hours for 2 days

9o. In the event Melissa received activated charcoal prior to admission, the initial dose of Mucomyst should be _____.

   A. unaltered
   B. doubled
   C. divided in half and administered 4 hours apart
   D. doubled, but given as 2 doses 4 hours apart

9p. The trade name for ondansetron is _____.

   A. Lotronex
   B. Zofran
   C. Kytril
   D. Anzemet

9q. Ondansetron is prescribed to Melissa for the treatment of _____.

    A. gastric ulcers
    B. nausea and vomiting
    C. acetaminophen toxicity
    D. hyperglycemia

9r. Melissa's ondansetron dose should be adjusted to _____.

    A. 0.05 mg/kg
    B. 0.1 mg/kg
    C. 0.15 mg/kg
    D. 0.2 mg/kg

CASE 10

PHYSICIAN ORDER

Patient Weight: 11 kg

Administer activated charcoal every 4 hours
Obtain carbamazepine concentration every 8 hours

Date/Time: 8/16/1345   **Patient Name:** Courtney Lipcomb
Physician: Anita Ling   **Patient ID #:** 985587

MEDICAL PROFILE

Patient: Courtney Lipcomb   **Patient Weight:** 11 kg   **Age:** 2 y/o

Present Illness: Carbamazepine ingestion of an unknown quantity of 100 mg tabs, possible seizure prior to admission

Medical History: Previously healthy

Labs: Na 140, K 3.9, Cl 101, C02 16, Cr 0.3, BUN 18, Glu 98, WBC 10,900, H/H 11.2/35.1, Plat 270,000, carbamazepine 28.5

PE: B/P 116/76, R 22, P 142, T 37.2 C

Cultures: Pending

Medication Profile:

10a. The trade name of carbamazepine is _____.

    A. Tegretol
    B. Tenormin
    C. Trental
    D. Timoptic

10b. Carbamazepine is primarily prescribed as a(n) _____.

    A. antihypertensive agent
    B. diuretic
    C. lipid-lowering agent
    D. anticonvulsant

10c. Which of the following mechanisms are associated with carbamazepine?

    A. Blockade of sodium channels
    B. Inhibition of acetylcholine receptors
    C. Inhibition of N-methyl-D-aspartate receptors
    D. A and B only
    E. A, B, and C

10d. Which of the following represents accepted therapeutic concentrations of carbamazepine?

    A. 2–8 mcg/mL
    B. 4–12 mcg/mL
    C. 5–15 mcg/mL
    D. 10–20 mcg/mL

10e. Which of the following is a potential manifestation of carbamazepine toxicity?

    A. Cardiac arrhythmias
    B. Respiratory depression
    C. Seizures
    D. A and B only
    E. A, B, and C

10f. The metabolite of carbamazepine that shares therapeutic and toxic effects with the parent compound is _____.

    A. 5-hydroxy-carbamazepine
    B. carbamazepine-10, 11-epoxide
    C. carbamazepine-5, 10-phenol
    D. 10-hydroxy-carbamazepine

10g. In the presence of an overdose, which is true regarding carbamazepine?

    A. Absorption is often slow and erratic
    B. Cardiovascular sodium channels are minimally affected
    C. Peristalsis is increased
    D. A and B only
    E. A, B, and C

10h. In the event Courtney's seizure activity resumed, which of the following would be the most appropriate therapy to initiate?

    A. Lorazepam
    B. Phenytoin
    C. Carbatrol
    D. A and B only
    E. A, B, and C

10i. What would be an appropriate dose of activated charcoal to prescribe to Courtney?

    A. 500 mg/kg
    B. 5 gms/kg
    C. 30 gms
    D. 50 gms

10j. Which of the following is an important consideration when prescribing activated charcoal for Courtney?

    A. Only a single dose should be prescribed as multiple doses of activated charcoal have not proven beneficial subsequent to carbamazepine ingestions
    B. Gastrointestinal motility should be monitored closely
    C. Each dose of activated charcoal should be provided in a sorbitol base
    D. A and C only
    E. A, B, and C

10k. Which of the following is true regarding activated charcoal administration?

    A. Should be mixed aggressively with at least 240 mLs of water or milk and swallowed quickly before settling occurs
    B. Causes the stools to turn green
    C. Should be used cautiously in obtunded patients because of the risk of aspiration
    D. A and C only
    E. A, B, and C

10l. Approximately how many milliliters of activated charcoal (25 gm/120 mLs) should be prescribed to provide a dose of 10,000 milligrams?

    A. 20 mL
    B. 30 mL
    C. 40 mL
    D. 50 mL

CASE 11

PHYSICIAN ORDER

Patient Weight: 15 kg

Begin tobramycin 2 mg/kg iv q 8 h
Peak and trough with 3rd dose

Date/Time: 1/29/1600   **Patient Name:** John Highes
Physician: Jeff Haskell   **Patient ID #:** 785587

MEDICAL PROFILE

Patient: John Highes   **Patient Weight:** 15 kg   **Age:** 3 y/o

Present Illness: Respiratory distress, pneumonia

Medical History: Unremarkable

Labs: Na 140, K 3.7, Cl 105, C02 28, Cr 0.4, BUN 3, Glu 187, Ca 8.5, ICA 1.16, Mg 1.4, WBC 20900, H/H 9.9/28.3, Plat 174,000, Segs 41%, Bands 31%, Lymphs 3%, Monos 2%, CRP 12.4, Lactate 1.8, Phos 4.5, Alk Phos 68, ALT 15, AST 27, Alb 3.6

Vitals: B/P 70/46, R 18, P 88, T 39 C

Cultures: Preliminary result: Possible *Staphylococcus* and *Pseudomonas* (Tracheal)

Medication Profile:

Date	Medication
1/28/1900	Vancomycin 300 mg iv q 8 h
1/28/1900	Zosyn 1250 mg iv q 6 h
1/29/0200	Fentanyl 30 mcg/hr
1/29/0200	Lorazepam 1.5 mg/hr
1/29/0200	Vecuronium 1.5 mg/hr
1/29/0200	Dopamine 15 mcg/kg/hr
1/29/0200	Ranitidine 15 mg iv q 8 h

11a. Which of John's laboratory values needs to be corrected?

   A. Sodium
   B. Potassium
   C. Ionized calcium
   D. Magnesium

11b. Which of John's reported laboratory values is consistent with a diagnosis of a bacterial infection?

   A. WBC
   B. CRP
   C. Bands
   D. A and C only
   E. A, B, and C

11c. Zosyn is a combination product consisting of
_____.

A. ticarcillin and clavulanate
B. ticarcillin and tazobactam
C. piperacillin and clavulanate
D. piperacillin and tazobactam

11d. Zosyn provides antibacterial coverage against
_____.

A. gram-negative aerobes
B. gram-positive aerobes
C. anaerobes
D. A and B only
E. A, B, and C

11e. Which of the following antibiotics provides a similar spectrum of antimicrobial activity to that of Zosyn?

A. Timentin
B. Claforan
C. Ceftin
D. Rocephin

11f. Which of John's medications is improperly dosed?

A. Fentanyl
B. Vancomycin
C. Lorazepam
D. Dopamine

11g. A vancomycin peak and trough concentration were reported as 28 and 7 mcg/mL at 1300 and 1900, respectively. What is the calculated half-life of vancomycin?

A. 2 hours
B. 3 hours
C. 4 hours
D. 6 hours

11h. At low doses (i.e., 1–5 mcg/kg/min), dopamine predominately affects which type of receptor?

A. α-1
B. β-1
C. β-2
D. Dopaminergic

11i. The vasoconstrictive effects of dopamine are predominately a result of its interaction with which receptor type?

A. α-1
B. β-1
C. β-2
D. Dopaminergic

11j. As opposed to intermittent dosing, dopamine is administered via continuous infusion because of
_____.

A. increased adverse effects resulting from intermittent dosing
B. its rapid terminal elimination half-life
C. its prolonged distribution phase
D. B and C only

11k. Which of the following is a trade name for dopamine?

A. Dobutrex
B. Inocor
C. Intropin
D. Primacor

11l. Which of the following medications is the drug of choice for the treatment of dopamine extravasation?

A. Phenylephrine
B. Phentolamine
C. Hyaluronidase
D. Mannitol

11m. A more appropriate initial tobramycin regimen for John would be _____.

A. 15 mg iv q 8 h
B. 30 mg iv q 8 h
C. 40 mg iv q 8 h
D. 45 mg iv q 8 h

11n. Tobramycin was mainly prescribed to John to provide additional antimicrobial coverage against
_____.

A. gram-positive bacteria
B. gram-negative bacteria
C. anaerobes
D. atypical bacteria

11o. The most appropriate targeted serum peak and trough concentrations of tobramycin for John would include which of the following?

A. Peak 8–12 mcg/mL, trough > 2 mcg/mL
B. Peak 8–12 mcg/mL, trough < 2 mcg/mL
C. Peak 5–10 mcg/mL, trough 1–2 mcg/mL
D. Peak 5–10 mcg/mL, trough < 2 mcg/mL

11p. Peak and trough concentrations are requested with John's third tobramycin dose because _____.

    A. accurate pharmacokinetic calculations cannot be performed on the first or second dose

    B. steady-state concentrations will most likely occur by the third dose

    C. obtaining concentrations on the third dose is more convenient for the nursing staff

    D. A and B only

CASE 12

PHYSICIAN ORDER

Patient Weight: 19 kg

Sodium phosphate 0.2 mMol/kg iv
Timentin 1500 mg iv q 6 h
Calcium gluconate 1.9 gms iv over 1 hour

Date/Time: 8/6/0900
Physician: Bill Richards

Patient Name: Seth Haskell
Patient ID #: 845587

MEDICAL PROFILE

Patient: Seth Haskell   **Patient Weight:** 19 kg   **Age:** 4 y/o

Present Illness: Septic shock, respiratory distress, intubated, mechanical ventilation

Medical History: Seizures

Labs: Na 144, K 3.3, Cl 99, C02 29, Cr 0.3, BUN 8, Glu 112, ICA 0.98, Mg 1.9, WBC 19000, H/H 10.8/29.5, Plat 391,000, Segs 64%, Bands 22%, CRP 15, Phos 1.9, Ammonia 80, Alk Phos 153, ALT 33, AST 36, Valproic acid 90

Vitals: B/P 68/46, R 18, P 80, T 39.5 C

Cultures: Blood: Staph species; Tracheal: *Pseudomonas*—sensitive to gentamicin, ceftazidime, tobramycin, piperacillin, imipenem, and ticarcillin

Medication Profile:

Date	Medication
8/5/1500	Lorazepam 2 mg/hr
8/5/1500	Fentanyl 20 mcg/hr
8/5/1500	Vecuronium 2 mg/hr
8/5/1300	Dopamine 20 mcg/kg/min
8/5/1300	Norepinephrine 0.008 mcg/kg/min
8/5/1200	Vancomycin 400 mg iv q 8 h
8/5/1200	Gentamicin 50 mg iv q 8 h
8/5/1200	Ceftazidime 1 gm iv q 6 h
8/5/1200	Ranitidine 20 mg iv q 8 h
8/5/1200	Valproic acid 250 mg iv q 8 h

12a. The trade name for norepinephrine is
_____.

    A. Adrenalin
    B. Levophed
    C. Primacor
    D. Nitropress

12b. Norepinephrine administration results in significant vasoconstriction resulting from it primarily stimulating _____ receptors.

    A. α-1
    B. α-2
    C. β-1
    D. β-2

12c. Which of the following is a benefit of norepinephrine in the treatment of septic shock?

    A. Attenuation of inappropriate vasodilatation
    B. Attenuation of myocardial depression
    C. Improvement of renal perfusion pressure
    D. A and B only
    E. A, B, and C

12d. Potential adverse effects from norepinephrine include _____.

    A. hypertension
    B. sweating
    C. arrhythmias
    D. A and C only
    E. A, B, and C

12e. A more appropriate norepinephrine regimen for Seth would be _____.

    A. 0.08 mcg/kg/min
    B. 0.8 mcg/kg/hr
    C. 8 mcg/kg/min
    D. 8 mcg/kg/hr

12f. In the event that maximum recommended doses of norepinephrine and dopamine fail to correct Seth's hypotensive state, which of the following laboratory values might prove useful in providing alternative therapy?

    A. Albumin
    B. Cortisol
    C. Epinephrine
    D. Hemoglobin

12g. Which of Seth's medications may increase his risk of adverse effects associated with vecuronium?

    A. Fentanyl
    B. Gentamicin
    C. Albuterol
    D. Norepinephrine

12h. Which of the following techniques may be used to minimize the risk of vecuronium-induced adverse effects?

    A. Only use concurrent sedative agents when necessary
    B. Regularly assess train of four response
    C. Use concurrent diuretic therapy to enhance elimination
    D. A and B only
    E. A, B, and C

12i. Which of the following medications would be an alternative for vecuronium?

    A. Propofol
    B. Pentobarbital
    C. Lorazepam
    D. Pancuronium

12j. In the event that Seth developed renal and or hepatic failure, which of the following would be the most appropriate alternative to vecuronium?

    A. Mivacurium
    B. Rocuronium
    C. Doxacurium
    D. Cisatracurium

12k. Timentin is a combination product containing _____.

    A. piperacillin and tazobactam
    B. ticarcillin and clavulanate
    C. ampicillin and sulbactam
    D. amoxicillin and clavulanic acid

12l. With the addition of Timentin to Seth's profile, which of his current medications should be discontinued?

    A. Vancomycin
    B. Ceftazidime
    C. Gentamicin
    D. A and B only
    E. A, B, and C

12m. The trade name for the injectable form of valproic acid is _____.

A. Depakote
B. Depakene
C. Depacon
D. Dilantin

12n. The therapeutic range for valproic acid for the majority of patients is _____ mcg/mL.

A. 5–15
B. 10–20
C. 15–40
D. 50–100

12o. In lieu of sodium phosphate, it would have been more prudent to prescribe _____ for Seth.

A. potassium phosphate
B. magnesium phosphate
C. calcium phosphate
D. aluminum phosphate

12p. How many milliequivalents of sodium will Seth receive with the prescribed dose of sodium phosphate?

A. 1.9 mEq
B. 3.8 mEq
C. 5.1 mEq
D. 7.5 mEq

12q. Seth's sodium phosphate dose should be infused over a minimum of _____.

A. 0.5–1 hour
B. 1–2 hours
C. 4–6 hours
D. 6–12 hours

12r. Which of Seth's medications would most likely be implicated for his altered ammonia serum concentration?

A. Dopamine
B. Valproic Acid
C. Norepinephrine
D. Lorazepam

12s. Which of the following is prescribed for the treatment of hyperammonemia?

A. Gentamicin
B. Lactulose
C. Ascorbic acid
D. A and B only
E. A, B, and C

12t. Calcium gluconate for injection is available as a 10% solution. How many milliliters are needed to provide Seth with his prescribed dose?

A. 1.9 mL
B. 3.8 mL
C. 19 mL
D. 38 mL

12u. One gram of calcium gluconate contains 90 mg (4.5 mEq) of elemental calcium. How many milliequivalents of elemental calcium will Seth receive from his prescribed dose?

A. 4.5 mEq
B. 8.6 mEq
C. 9 mEq
D. 10 mEq

CASE 13

PHYSICIAN ORDER

Patient Weight: 11 kg

Dexamethasone 1.1 mg iv q 6 hours × 2 days
Ranitidine 10 mg iv q 8 h

Date/Time: 9/5/1600
Physician: Greg Green

Patient Name: William Phillips
Patient ID #: 695587

MEDICAL PROFILE

Patient: William Phillips

Patient Weight: 11 kg   **Age:** 8 m/o

Present Illness: R/O meningitis

Medical History: Previously healthy

Labs: Na 141, K 4.8, Cl 113, C02 21.6, Cr 0.4, BUN 8, Glu 107, Ca 9.2, Mg 2.1, WBC 9400, H/H 11.3/32.9, Plat 240,000, Segs 23%, Bands 12%, CRP 8

Cultures: CSF: WBC 2170 mm^3, PMN 80%, Protein 220, Glucose 30

Medication Profile:

Date	Medication
9/5/1400	Cefotaxime 1 gm iv q 8 h
9/5/1400	Acetaminophen 100 mg po q 4 h prn

13a. Which of the following is a sign of meningitis?

   A. Fever
   B. Neck stiffness
   C. Photophobia
   D. A and B only
   E. A, B, and C

13b. Flexion of a patient's neck resulting in hip and knee flexion is termed _____ sign.

   A. Kernig's
   B. Brudzinski's
   C. Reye's
   D. meningitic

13c. In the absence of infection, which of the following is consistent with the composition of the cerebral spinal fluid?

   A. Protein content < 50 mg/dL
   B. Glucose concentration 30% of the serum glucose concentration
   C. White blood cells > 5 per mm^3
   D. A and B only
   E. A, B, and C

13d. Which of William's labs are consistent with bacterial meningitis?

   A. CSF protein
   B. CSF glucose
   C. CSF PMN's
   D. A and B only
   E. A, B, and C

13e. Patients diagnosed with bacterial meningitis typically present with CSF leukocyte counts between _____ mm^3.

   A. 10–100
   B. 10–1000
   C. 100–1000
   D. 100–10,000

13f. The most commonly identified cause of bacterial meningitis is _____.

   A. *Streptococcus pneumoniae*
   B. *Haemophilus influenzae*
   C. *Neisseria meningitides*
   D. *Listeria monocytogenes*

13g. The brand name of cefotaxime is _____.

   A. Claforan
   B. Ceftin
   C. Mefoxin
   D. Rocephin

13h. Cefotaxime is classified as a _____ generation cephalosporin.

   A. first-
   B. second-
   C. third-
   D. fourth-

13i. William's cefotaxime dose should be changed to _____.

   A. 500 mg iv q 6 h
   B. 750 mg iv q 8 h
   C. 800 mg iv q 6 h
   D. 1000 mg iv q 6 h

13j. Which of the following would be the most reasonable alternative for cefotaxime for William?

   A. Cefuroxime
   B. Ceftriaxone
   C. Ampicillin
   D. Ceftazidime

13k. Which of the following antibiotics would be prudent to prescribe to William?

   A. Vancomycin
   B. Chloramphenicol
   C. Ampicillin
   D. Gentamicin

13l. What is the rationale for prescribing dexamethasone to William?

   A. Provide protection against sensorineural hearing loss
   B. Modulate the enhanced meningeal inflammatory response
   C. Enhance the absorption of antibiotics across the blood-brain barrier
   D. A and B only
   E. A, B, and C

13m. William's dexamethasone order should be changed to _____.

   A. 1.1 mg iv q 8 hours
   B. 1.7 mg iv q 8 hours
   C. 1.7 mg iv q 6 hours
   D. 3.4 mg iv q 6 hours

13n. For optimal effects, William's first dexamethasone dose should be administered _____.

   A. prior to his first dose of cefotaxime
   B. as a 30-minute infusion to provide initial concentrations for a prolonged period of time
   C. 30 minutes after his first dose of cefotaxime
   D. A and B only
   E. B and C only

13o. Dexamethasone is available as a 4 mg/mL solution for injection. How many milliliters are needed to provide William's prescribed daily dose?

   A. 0.28 mL
   B. 0.56 mL
   C. 1.1 mL
   D. 2.2 mL

13p. Ranitidine was most likely prescribed for William to _____.

   A. prevent gastrointestinal adverse effects from dexamethasone
   B. enhance the absorption of cefotaxime
   C. provide an alkaline environment to assist in CSF bacterial destruction
   D. enhance the absorption of dexamethasone

CASE 14

PHYSICIAN ORDER

Patient Weight: <u>7.5 kg</u>

Ribavirin 6 gms daily for 5 days

Date/Time: <u>1/4/0900</u>
Physician: <u>Lang Pauley</u>

Patient Name: <u>Joe Nell</u>
Patient ID #: <u>897887</u>

MEDICAL PROFILE

Patient: Joe Nell

Patient Weight: 7.5 kg   **Age:** 1 y/o

Present Illness: RSV, respiratory distress

Medical History: BPD, multiple admissions for RSV

Labs: Na 137, K 5.5, Cl 105, C02 19.8, Cr 0.3, BUN 9, Glu 84, ICA 1.12, Mg 2.2, WBC 16400, H/H 12.2/35.8, Plat 345,000, Segs 40%, Bands 4%, CRP 2.4, Phos 4.8

Cultures: Nasopharyngeal – RSV; Endotracheal – gram-positive cocci

Medication Profile:

Date	Medication
1/4/0600	Ceftriaxone 400 mg iv q 8 h
1/4/0400	Albuterol 1.25 mg neb q 2 h
1/4/0400	Atrovent 250 mcg neb q 4 h
1/4/0400	Racemic epinephrine neb 0.4 ml q 2 h
1/4/0400	Methylprednisolone 8 mg iv q 6 h
1/4/0400	Ranitidine 8 mg iv q 8 h
1/4/0400	Fentanyl 7.5 mcg/hr
1/4/0400	Lorazepam 0.8 mg/hr
1/4/0400	Vecuronium 0.8 mg/hr

14a. Which of the following is true of respiratory syncytial virus (RSV)?

   A. Is an enveloped double-stranded virus
   B. Its G-protein functions to allow physical attachment of the virus to cells
   C. RSV A-infections are generally less severe than RSV B-infections
   D. B and C only
   E. A, B, and C

14b. Which of the following is true regarding the spread of RSV?

   A. The major inoculation sites are the eyes and mouth
   B. RSV-infected nasal secretions remain infectious on countertops for more than 6 hours
   C. RSV viral shedding only occurs for ∼ 3 to 5 days
   D. A and B only
   E. A, B, and C

14c. By 2 years of age, what percentage of infants will have been infected with RSV?

A. 10%
B. 30%
C. 50%
D. ~ 100%

14d. Which of the following is a potential sign/symptom associated with RSV?

A. Cough
B. Wheezing
C. Apnea
D. A and B only
E. A, B, and C

14e. Infants with which of the following conditions are at greatest risk of requiring hospitalization due to RSV?

A. Congenital heart disease
B. Bronchopulmonary dysplasia
C. Prematurity
D. B and C only
E. A, B, and C

14f. Which of Joe's aerosols will most likely be beneficial in the treatment of his RSV?

A. Albuterol
B. Atrovent
C. Racemic epinephrine
D. A and B only

14g. Which of the following is true regarding the administration of nebulized albuterol and Atrovent?

A. Albuterol and Atrovent solutions may be combined and administered together
B. Albuterol should be administered 15 minutes prior to Atrovent
C. Atrovent should be administered 15 minutes prior to albuterol
D. Albuterol and Atrovent should never be administered within 2 hours of one another

14h. The trade name for racemic epinephrine is _____.

A. Vaponefrin
B. Velban
C. Vasodilan
D. Vascor

14i. The recommended nebulized dose of racemic epinephrine is _____.

A. 0.05 mg/kg, not to exceed 0.5 mg
B. 0.05 ml/kg, not to exceed 0.5 mL
C. 0.5 mg/kg, not to exceed 0.5 mg
D. 0.5 ml/kg, not to exceed 0.5 mL

14j. Infants diagnosed with RSV should always receive which of the following therapies?

A. Supportive care
B. Corticosteroids
C. Ribavirin
D. A and B only
E. A, B, and C

14k. The trade name of ribavirin is _____.

A. Virazole
B. Synagis
C. Respigam
D. Cytogam

14l. Which of the following is true of ribavirin?

A. Is a broad spectrum virucidal agent
B. Is theoretically more effective when administered early in the course of the RSV infection
C. Is a human teratogen
D. A and C only
E. A, B, and C

14m. Ribavirin is administered via _____.

A. continuous intravenous infusion
B. intermittent intravenous boluses
C. small particle aerosol generator
D. total parenteral nutrition

14n. Joe's ribavirin dose should be administered as _____.

A. 6 grams over 18 hours
B. 2 grams over 2 hours three times a day
C. Either A or B
D. Neither A or B

14o. Possible adverse effects associated with ribavirin include _____.

A. bronchospasm
B. rash
C. ventilator malfunctioning
D. A and B only
E. A, B, and C

CASE 15

PHYSICIAN ORDER

Patient Weight: <u>44 kg</u>

Meperidine 25 mg iv q 4 h prn

Date/Time: 1/5/0200
Physician: <u>Paul Smithey</u>

Patient Name: <u>Tiffany Stull</u>
Patient ID #: <u>836887</u>

MEDICAL PROFILE

Patient: Tiffany Stull

Patient Weight: 44 kg   **Age:** 12 y/o

Present Illness: Sickle cell crises

Medical History: Sickle cell disease

Labs: Na 134, K 3.2, Cl 95, C02 24, Cr 1.4, BUN 7, Glu 88, ICA 1.11, Mg 2.1, WBC 12900, H/H 8.3/23.9, Plat 599,000, Phos 5.5, Alb 3.6

Vitals: B/P 133/53, P 88, R 20, T 38.2

Cultures: Pending

Medication Profile:

Date	Medication
1/5/0130	Ketorolac 25 mg iv q 6 h prn
1/5/0130	Cefuroxime 1500 mg iv q 8 h

15a. Acute sickle cell pain may be provoked by
_____.

   A. temperature extremes
   B. physical stress
   C. infections
   D. A and C only
   E. A, B, and C

15b. Acute sickle cell pain most commonly occurs in which of the following sites?

   A. Lower back
   B. Chest
   C. Thigh
   D. A and B only
   E. A, B, and C

15c. Sickle cell pain is due to _____.

   A. tissue ischemia caused by occlusion of vascular beds
   B. reperfusion to damaged vascular beds
   C. oxygenation of sickle hemoglobin
   D. oxygenation of hemoglobin S polymers

15d. The preferred class of analgesics for the treatment of acute sickle cell pain is the _____.

   A. parenteral opiates
   B. oral opiates
   C. parenteral nonsteroidal anti-inflammatory agents
   D. oral nonsteroidal anti-inflammatory agents

15e. Analgesics for acute sickle cell pain should be administered _____.

A. on an as-needed basis
B. scheduled around the clock
C. scheduled around the clock for the first 24 hours and then as needed
D. only via patient-controlled analgesia infusion pumps

15f. The trade name for meperidine is _____.

A. MS Contin
B. Demerol
C. Dilaudid
D. Oxycontin

15g. A more appropriate meperidine regimen for the treatment of acute sickle cell pain in a 44-kg patient would be _____.

A. 25 mg po q 4 h
B. 25 mg iv q 4 h
C. 50 mg iv q 4 h
D. 50 mg iv q 4 h prn

15h. The metabolite of meperidine that is commonly associated with seizure activity is _____.

A. 5-hydroxy-meperidine
B. normeperidine
C. 10,11–meperidine epoxide
D. 4-hydroxy-meperidine

15i. In lieu of meperidine, which of the following would be a more appropriate analgesic to prescribe to Tiffany?

A. Morphine
B. Naproxen
C. Fentanyl
D. A and C only
E. A, B, and C

15j. An equivalent dose of morphine to the dose of meperidine prescribed to Tiffany would be ~ _____ mg.

A. 3.5
B. 5
C. 7.5
D. 10

15k. The trade name for ketorolac is _____.

A. Orudis
B. Voltaren
C. Toradol
D. Miltown

15l. Ketorolac is classified as a(n) _____.

A. opiate
B. NSAID
C. phenothiazine
D. antiemetic

15m. Adverse effects associated with ketorolac therapy include _____.

A. renal impairment
B. GI bleeding
C. inhibition of platelet aggregation
D. B and C only
E. A, B, and C

15n. Which of the following actions is most appropriate with respect to Tiffany's ketorolac regimen?

A. Prescribed dose should be administered every 6 hours
B. Regimen should be changed to 25 mg iv q 8 hours
C. Regimen should be changed to 30 mg iv q 6 hours
D. Should be discontinued

15o. Ketorolac is available as a(n) _____ preparation.

A. parenteral
B. oral
C. ophthalmic
D. A and B only
E. A, B, and C

15p. It is recommended that ketorolac use should not exceed _____ days.

A. 5
B. 7
C. 10
D. 14

CASE 16

PHYSICIAN ORDER

Patient Weight: 55 kg

Humulin N 10 u/hr

Date/Time: 3/13/0900
Physician: Jeff Swaim

Patient Name: Nell Stokes
Patient ID #: 693887

MEDICAL PROFILE

Patient: Nell Stokes   **Patient Weight:** 55 kg   **Age:** 16 y/o

Present Illness: DKA

Medical History: Type I Diabetes

Labs: Na 136, K 5.7, Cl 107, C02 5, Cr 1.3, BUN 18, Glu 504, ICA 1.22, Mg 2.7, WBC 24200, H/H 15.1/43.2, Plat 455,000, Segs 60%, Bands 5%, Phos 5.4, Ketones 4+

Urinalysis: Specific gravity 1.025, pH 5, protein 30, glucose +, Ketones > 80

Medication Profile:

Date	Medication
3/13/0845	Acetaminophen 500 mg po q 4 h prn
3/13/0700	0.9% saline 1000 mL over 60 minutes

16a. Which of the following is a characteristic of diabetic ketoacidosis (DKA)?

    A. Serum glucose > 250 mg/dL
    B. Arterial blood pH > 7.3
    C. Serum bicarbonate > 15 mEq/L
    D. A and B only
    E. A, B, and C

16b. In a patient previously diagnosed with diabetes, precipitating events leading to DKA include _____.

    A. noncompliance with insulin therapy
    B. infections
    C. psychological stress
    D. A and B only
    E. A, B, and C

16c. The most common cause of death in patients presenting with DKA is _____.

    A. hypokalemia
    B. cerebral edema
    C. metabolic acidosis
    D. dehydration

16d. Which of Nell's laboratory values is consistent with DKA?

    A. Potassium
    B. WBC
    C. Ketones
    D. B and C only
    E. A, B, and C

16e. Which of Nell's urinalysis values is consistent with DKA?

A. Specific gravity
B. Glucose
C. Ketones
D. B and C only
E. A, B, and C

16f. The most important aspect in the initial management of a patient presenting with DKA is providing _____therapy.

A. insulin
B. hydration
C. electrolyte
D. bicarbonate

16g. Nell was initially prescribed normal saline because _____.

A. DKA patients are invariably dehydrated
B. isotonic saline is restricted to the intracellular fluid space and rapidly corrects plasma volume
C. isotonic saline is similar to fluid lost during osmotic diuresis
D. A and B only
E. A, B, and C

16h. Following Nell's fluid bolus with normal saline, her subsequent intravenous fluid will most likely be _____.

A. 0.9% saline
B. 0.45% saline
C. 3% saline
D. D5W

16i. Which of the following is true regarding additives and the initial fluid replacement of patients presenting with DKA?

A. Potassium is routinely added to the initial fluid
B. Phosphate is routinely added to the initial fluid
C. Neither potassium nor phosphate is routinely added to the initial fluid
D. Both A and B

16j. Which of the following is true regarding bicarbonate in the treatment of patients with DKA?

A. Is routinely prescribed to resolve the associated metabolic acidosis
B. Should only be considered when the arterial pH is greater than 7.0
C. May precipitate hypokalemia
D. B and C only
E. A, B, and C

16k. Which of the following insulin products should be substituted for the one prescribed for Nell?

A. Ultralente
B. Lente
C. Humulin R
D. Humulin 70/30

16l. The correct dose of insulin for Nell is _____ units/hr.

A. 2.75
B. 5.5
C. 7
D. 8.25

16m. Insulin is supplied in a concentration of 100 units/mL. How many milliliters are needed to provide Nell with her prescribed dose for 24 hours?

A. 0.024 mL
B. 0.24 mL
C. 2.4 mL
D. 24 mL

16n. The effect of insulin administration on serum potassium is _____.

A. reentry of potassium into the intracellular compartment
B. reentry of potassium into the extracellular compartment
C. elevated potassium concentrations resulting from enhanced renal tubular absorption
D. decreased potassium concentrations as a result of increased protein binding

16o. During the administration of insulin therapy, Nell's serum glucose falls below 200 mg/dL. Which of the following interventions would be most appropriate?

A. Decrease the insulin dose by 25%
B. Decrease the insulin dose by 50%
C. Discontinue the insulin infusion for 1 hour and then resume at the same dose.
D. Add 5–10% dextrose to her current maintenance fluids

CASE 17

PHYSICIAN ORDER

Patient Weight: <u>4.5 kg</u>

Milrinone 0.375 mcg/kg/hr
Ketorolac 2.5 mg iv q 6 h
Calcium Carbonate 100 mg iv × 1 dose

Date/Time: <u>8/15/1400</u>   **Patient Name:** <u>Daniel Stone</u>
Physician: <u>Joe Tiswell</u>   **Patient ID #:** <u>363887</u>

MEDICAL PROFILE

Patient: Daniel Stone   **Patient Weight:** 4.5 kg   **Age:** 4 m/o

Present Illness: Hypoplastic left heart, post-op

Medical History: Coarctation of the aorta

Labs: Na 144, K 3.1, Cl 89, C02 32, Cr 0.7, BUN 14, Glu 121, ICA 1.06, Mg 1.9, WBC 11300, H/H 15.9/45.9, Plat 110,000

Vitals: B/P 100/60, P 166, R 20

Medication Profile:

Date	Medication
8/15/1300	Dopamine 10 mcg/kg/min
8/15/1300	Nitroprusside 1 mcg/kg/min
8/15/1300	Furosemide 1 mg/hr
8/15/1300	Morphine 0.2 mg iv q 3 h prn
8/15/1300	Cefazolin 150 mg iv q 8 h x 6 doses
8/15/1300	Ranitidine 5 mg iv q 8 h

17a. Which of the following is true regarding hypoplastic left heart syndrome?

   A. Is the most common cause of death from cardiac defects during the first month of life
   B. Coarctation of the aorta is a common concurrent finding
   C. A ventricular septal defect may also be present
   D. B and C only
   E. A, B, and C

17b. Which of the following surgical procedures might be performed in Daniel?

   A. Norwood
   B. Fontan
   C. Glenn
   D. A and B only
   E. A, B, and C

17c. Daniel's laboratory values are consistent with a
_____.

   A. furosemide-induced metabolic alkalosis
   B. furosemide-induced metabolic acidosis
   C. dopamine-induced metabolic alkalosis
   D. dopamine-induced metabolic acidosis

17d. Which of the following should also be prescribed
for Daniel?

   A. Potassium chloride
   B. Magnesium sulfate
   C. Sodium chloride
   D. Potassium acetate

17e. Daniel's calcium order should be rewritten as

_____.

   A. Calcium carbonate 450 mg iv $\times$ 1 dose
   B. Calcium gluconate 450 mg iv $\times$ 1 dose
   C. Calcium chloride 450 mg iv $\times$ 1 dose
   D. Calcium chloride 1 gm iv $\times$ 1 dose

17f. A desired ionized calcium concentration in Daniel
would be _____ mMol/L.

   A. 1.05
   B. 1.12
   C. 1.9
   D. 2.5

17g. How many milligrams of dopamine per 100
milliliters of diluent would be necessary to provide
Daniel with his prescribed dose given an infusion
rate of 2 mL/hr and an "N" factor of 5?

   A. 65 mg
   B. 100 mg
   C. 135 mg
   D. 200 mg

17h. The brand name for nitroprusside is _____.

   A. Nitrogard
   B. Nitropress
   C. Nitro-Dur
   D. Nitrostat

17i. Nitroprusside is classified as a _____.

   A. diuretic
   B. vasodilator
   C. vasoconstrictor
   D. calcium antagonist

17j. Patients receiving nitroprusside for prolonged
periods of time are at risk for _____ toxicity.

   A. sodium
   B. cyanide
   C. benzyl alcohol
   D. propylene glycol

17k. To prevent toxicity, nitroprusside may be mixed
with _____.

   A. sodium thiosulfate
   B. sodium thiocyanate
   C. sodium thiocyanide
   D. sodium thiosulfide

17l. Which of the following is true of nitroprusside?

   A. Solution should be wrapped with an opaque
material during administration
   B. A blue color indicates solution is stable and
may be administered
   C. Normal dosing range is 5–10 mcg/kg/min
   D. Is available in both oral and parenteral dosage
forms

17m. The trade name of milrinone is _____.

   A. Primacor
   B. Inocor
   C. Dobutrex
   D. Adrenalin

17n. Milrinone is most closely related to _____.

   A. amrinone
   B. nitroprusside
   C. dopamine
   D. dobutamine

17o. Compared with its predecessor, which of the
following adverse effects occur less often with
milrinone?

   A. Hypotension
   B. Hypertension
   C. Thrombocytopenia
   D. Histamine release

17p. Which of the following is true of milrinone?

   A. Is primarily metabolized by monoamine oxidase
   B. Half-life is similar to that of pressor agents
such as dopamine and norepinephrine
   C. Is beneficial to patients with β-adrenergic
dysfunction
   D. A and C only
   E. A, B, and C

17q. A more appropriate dose of milrinone for Daniel would be a _____.

A. loading dose of 50 mcg/kg, followed by 0.375 mcg/kg/hr
B. loading dose of 50 mcg/kg, followed by 0.375 mcg/kg/min
C. loading dose of 50 mg/kg, followed by 0.375 mg/kg/hr
D. loading dose of 50 mg/kg, followed by 0.375 mg/kg/min

17r. Daniel's ketorolac order should be modified to _____.

A. 2.5 mg iv q 8 h
B. 2.5 mg iv q 6 h prn
C. 2.5 mg iv q 8 h prn
D. 2.5 mg iv q 6 h × 24 hours

CASE 18

PHYSICIAN ORDER

Patient Weight: 5 kg

Propranolol 0.05 mg/kg iv push

Date/Time: 1/5/0200
Physician: Andre Johnson

Patient Name: Ben Stokes
Patient ID #: 583887

MEDICAL PROFILE

Patient: Ben Stokes   **Patient Weight:** 5 kg   **Age:** 4 m/o

Present Illness: Cyanotic spell

Medical History: TOF

Labs: Na 137, K 3.4, Cl 101, C02 17, Cr 0.6, BUN 12, Glu 109, ICA 1.32, Mg 1.9, WBC 14300, H/H 9.9/29, Plat 147,000

Vitals: B/P 70/40, P 160, R 60, T 37.5

Medication Profile:

Date	Medication
1/5/0130	Morphine sulfate 0.2 mg/kg iv prn
1/5/0130	Sodium bicarbonate 1 mEq/kg iv x 2 if needed

18a. Ben's congenital anomaly most likely includes
_____.

   A. a large VSD
   B. RV outflow tract obstruction
   C. an overriding of the aorta
   D. A and B only
   E. A, B, and C

18b. Which of the following is likely to be present in Ben?

   A. Heart murmur
   B. Cyanosis
   C. Hyperpnea
   D. B and C only
   E. A, B, and C

18c. Ben was most likely prescribed morphine sulfate because of its _____ effects.

   A. analgesic
   B. respiratory depressant
   C. sedative
   D. anti-inflammatory

18d. In the absence of intravenous access, morphine sulfate may also be administered _____.

   A. intramuscularly
   B. subcutaneously
   C. orally
   D. A and C only
   E. A, B, and C

18e. How many milliliters of an 8.4% bicarbonate solution for injection are needed to provide Ben with his prescribed dose? (1 mEq sodium bicarbonate = 84 mg)

A. 5 mL
B. 8.4 mL
C. 12 mL
D. 16 mL

18f. Which of the following is true regarding sodium bicarbonate?

A. Dissociates to provide bicarbonate ion which neutralizes hydrogen ion concentrations
B. Caution is warranted when administered to patients with congestive heart failure
C. Because of its hypotonicity, tissue necrosis subsequent to extravasation is possible
D. A and B only
E. A, B, and C

18g. The trade name for propranolol is _____.

A. Visken
B. Inderal
C. Tenormin
D. Lopressor

18h. Propranolol is classified as a _____.

A. selective α-1 adrenergic antagonist
B. non-selective α-adrenergic antagonist
C. selective β-1 adrenergic antagonist
D. non-selective β-adrenergic antagonist

18i. The maximum recommended dose of intravenous propranolol for an infant, irrespective of weight, is _____.

A. 1 mg
B. 2 mg
C. 3 mg
D. 5 mg

18j. It is desired to prepare a 0.01% dilution of propranolol. How many milliliters of the dilution should be administered to provide Ben with his prescribed dose?

A. 0.5 mL
B. 1 mL
C. 2.5 mL
D. 5 mL

18k. Which of the following would be an alternative therapy to propranolol for the treatment of Ben's cyanotic spell?

A. Neo-Synephrine
B. Phenylephrine
C. Ketamine
D. A and B only
E. A, B, and C

18l. Which of the following would be most appropriate for prophylaxis for recurrent cyanotic spells?

A. Neo-Synephrine
B. Propranolol
C. Dopamine
D. Hydralazine

CASE 19

PHYSICIAN ORDER

Patient Weight: 3.5 kg

Decrease digoxin to 13 mcg iv q 12 h
Obtain digoxin concentration 2 hours after the third dose

Date/Time: 11/16/0900
Physician: Larry Wilson

Patient Name: James Duhn
Patient ID #: 693697

MEDICAL PROFILE

Patient: James Duhn

Patient Weight: 3.5 kg **Age:** 3 w/o

Present Illness: VSD, PDA, Interrupted aortic arch

Medical History: 39-weeks gestation

Labs: Na 145, K 3.1, Cl 100, C02 21.4, Cr 0.4, BUN 10, Glu 111, ICA 1.18, Mg 2.7, WBC 15700, H/H 11.5/33.7, Plat 218,000, Segs 58%, Bands 8%, Phos 5.5, Lactate 1.4, CRP 3.4, Phenobarbital 37, Digoxin 2.2

Vitals: B/P 66/35, P 134, R 68, T 37.0

Cultures: Endotrachael aspirate: Coagulase negative *Staphylococcus*

Medication Profile:

Date	Medication
11/14/0700	Prostin 1 mcg/kg/min
11/14/0700	Furosemide 3.5 mg iv q 6 h
11/14/0700	Digoxin 15 mcg iv q 12 h
11/14/0700	Phenobarbital 15 mg iv qd
11/14/0700	Dopamine 20 mcg/kg/min
11/15/1100	Spironolactone 3.5 mg po q 12 h
11/15/1900	Vancomycin 35 mg iv qd
11/15/1900	Ceftazidime 170 mg iv q 8 h

19a. Interrupted aortic arch is an extreme form of coarctation of the aorta and may also be associated with (a) _____.

    A. VSD
    B. PDA
    C. Di George syndrome
    D. A and B only
    E. A, B, and C

19b. Which of the following is true of a ventricular septal defect (VSD)?

    A. Is the least common form of congenital heart disease
    B. Infants with a small VSD are usually cyanotic and underdeveloped
    C. With a moderate to large VSD, delayed growth and development and congestive heart failure are relatively common during infancy
    D. Surgery is the primary form of treatment with drug therapy being reserved for nonsurgical candidates

19c. Digoxin is a _____.

    A. positive inotrope
    B. positive chronotrope
    C. negative chronotrope
    D. A and B only
    E. A and C only

19d. Which of the following effects might be expected given James' reported potassium concentration?

    A. Increased activity of digoxin
    B. Decreased activity of digoxin
    C. Increased activity of dopamine
    D. Decreased activity of dopamine

19e. Which of the following methods would be most appropriate in administering a loading dose of digoxin?

    A. Administer as a single dose over 5–10 minutes
    B. Administer 1/2 of the loading dose followed by the remainder divided equally and administered 8 hours apart
    C. Divide the loading dose in half and administer 6 hours apart
    D. Administer as three equal aliquots over 5–10 minutes 3 hours apart

19f. An accepted therapeutic serum concentration of digoxin is _____.

    A. 0.8–2 mcg/mL
    B. 0.8–2 ng/mL
    C. 0.5–3 mcg/mL
    D. 0.5–3 ng/mL

19g. Digoxin concentrations should be obtained either just prior to a dose (trough) or no sooner than _____ hour(s) after a dose.

    A. 1
    B. 2
    C. 3
    D. 6

19h. Which of the following dosage forms of digoxin has the greatest bioavailability?

    A. Tablets
    B. Capsules
    C. Liquid
    D. Both A and B have equal bioavailability

19i. The presence of endogenous digoxin-like substances may have altered James' digoxin concentration. In what patient population have these been identified?

    A. Pregnant patients
    B. Young children
    C. Patients with hepatic disease
    D. A and B only
    E. A, B, and C

19j. Instead of lowering James' digoxin dose, a more appropriate action would have been to _____.

    A. observe the patient for clinical signs of digoxin toxicity
    B. obtain a column-separated digoxin concentration
    C. discontinue the digoxin for 12 hours and recheck the concentration
    D. A and B only
    E. A, B, and C

19k. Digoxin is available as a 100 mcg/mL injectable pediatric dosage form. Which of the following would be the most appropriate technique for preparing James' digoxin dose?

   A. Obtain 0.13 mL of the stock solution
   B. Obtain 1.3 mLs of the stock solution
   C. Obtain 0.65 mLs of a digoxin dilution prepared by diluting 1 mL of stock solution to 5 mL with a diluent
   D. Obtain 0.65 mLs of a digoxin dilution prepared by diluting 1 mL of stock solution to 10 mL with a diluent

19l. The antidote for digoxin toxicity is _____.

   A. digoxin immune fab
   B. digitoxin
   C. deferoxamine
   D. desmopressin

19m. Which of the following would be a more appropriate dose of alprostadil for James?

   A. 0.01 mcg/kg/min
   B. 0.1 mcg/kg/min
   C. 0.01 mcg/kg/hr
   D. 0.1 mcg/kg/hr

19n. Which of the following medications is associated with hyperkalemia?

   A. Furosemide
   B. Spironolactone
   C. Digoxin
   D. Alprostadil

19o. Approximately, what is the equivalent oral dose of furosemide to the intravenous dose prescribed to James?

   A. 1.75 mg
   B. 3.5 mg
   C. 7 mg
   D. 10 mg

19p. Which of the following medications prescribed to James most likely warrants a dosage adjustment?

   A. Ceftazidime
   B. Phenobarbital
   C. Vancomycin
   D. Furosemide

19q. Based on James' cultures, which of the following medications might be discontinued?

   A. Alprostadil
   B. Spironolactone
   C. Vancomycin
   D. Ceftazidime

CASE 20

PHYSICIAN ORDER

Patient Weight: 7.5 kg

Increase continuous infusion of FK-506 to 0.3 mg/kg/day
Obtain FK-506 concentration in 48 hours

Date/Time: 5/28/0900   **Patient Name:** Chris Taap
Physician: James Shuler   **Patient ID #:** 793697

MEDICAL PROFILE

Patient: Chris Taap   **Patient Weight:** 7.5 kg   **Age:** 15 m/o

Present Illness: S/P liver transplant

Medical History: Biliary atresia, ascites, progressive liver failure

Labs: Na 144, K 3.5, Cl 97, C02 23, Cr 0.4, BUN 33, Glu 70, Mg 1.6, WBC 1700, H/H 9.1/28.2, Plat 56,000, Phos 3.9, Alb 3.3, Ca 8.4, Alk P 71, AST 77, ALT 108, GGT 64, D Bili 1.1, I Bili 1.7, Chol 109, TG 137, FK-506 (blood) 1.2

Vitals: B/P 146/77, P 80, R 16, T 36.2

Medication Profile:

Date	Medication
5/26/1000	FK-506 0.5 mg iv q 12 h continuous infusion
5/26/1000	Unasyn 350 mg iv q 6 h
5/26/1000	Acyclovir 35 mg iv qd
5/26/1000	Nystatin 2.5 mL ng q 6 h
5/26/0900	MVI pediatric iv qd
5/26/0900	Carafate 1 gm ng q 6 h
5/26/0900	Methylprednisolone 7.5 mg iv qd (tapering)
5/26/0900	Morphine 0.5–1 mg iv q 1 h prn
5/26/0900	Acetaminophen 100 mg pr q 4–6 h prn

20a. Chris' sucralfate dose should be adjusted to
_____.

    A. 100 mg po q 6 h
    B. 250 mg po q 6 h
    C. 500 mg po q 6 h
    D. 1000 mg po q 8 h

20b. Which of the following best describes sucralfate's mechanism of action?

    A. Antagonist
    B. Histamine-2 antagonist
    C. Proton pump inhibitor
    D. Mucosal protectant

20c. Unasyn is a combination product containing
_____.

A. piperacillin and tazobactam
B. piperacillin and sulbactam
C. ampicillin and sulbactam
D. ticarcillin and clavulanic acid

20d. Approximately how many milligrams of the major antibacterial component of Unasyn is Chris receiving with each dose?

A. 100 mg
B. 150 mg
C. 250 mg
D. 350 mg

20e. The trade name for FK-506 is _____.

A. Cellcept
B. Prograf
C. Neoral
D. Sandimmune

20f. FK-506 binds to immunophilins termed FK-binding proteins that in turn bind to and inhibit _____, of which is/are believed to mediate the immunosuppressive activity of FK-506.

A. T-Lymphocytes
B. tumor necrosis factor
C. calcineurin
D. macrophages

20g. Which of the following is true regarding the disposition of FK-506?

A. Absorption depends on the availability of bile acids
B. Oral bioavailability is ~ 90%
C. Is extensively metabolized by the liver
D. Is present in low concentrations in the lungs, spleen, and heart

20h. An accepted therapeutic blood concentration of FK-506 is _____.

A. 10–20 ng/mL
B. 10–20 mcg/mL
C. 0.5–2.0 ng/mL
D. 0.5–2.0 mcg/mL

20i. A reasonable initial dose of intravenous FK-506 for Chris would be _____.

A. 0.01 mg/kg/hr
B. 0.1 mg/kg/day
C. 0.3 mg/kg/hr
D. 0.1 mg/kg/hr

20j. A reasonable initial oral dose of FK-506 for a pediatric patient would be _____ mg/kg every 12 hours.

A. 0.05
B. 0.1
C. 0.15
D. 0.2

20k. Subsequent to Chris' dosage adjustment, which of the following would be the most appropriate time to obtain a follow-up FK-506 blood concentration?

A. 5 hours after beginning the infusion
B. 10 hours after beginning the infusion
C. 24 hours after beginning the infusion
D. As ordered, 48 hours after beginning the infusion

20l. Concurrent administration of which of the following medications may lead to increased FK-506 concentrations?

A. Diltiazem
B. Ketoconazole
C. Fluconazole
D. B and C only
E. A, B, and C

20m. Which of the following are potential complications from FK-506 administration?

A. Hypertension
B. Hyperglycemia
C. Hyperkalemia
D. A and B only
E. A, B, and C

20n. How many milliliters of FK-506 (5 mg/mL) are needed to provide Chris with a 12-hour supply of his newly prescribed dose?

A. 0.23 mL
B. 0.45 mL
C. 1.2 mL
D. 2.3 mL

20o. In the event Chris begins to exhibit signs of organ rejection, which of the following medications might he be prescribed?

A. OKT3
B. Additional corticosteroids
C. Azathioprine
D. A and B only
E. A, B, and C

20p. Which of the following is an immunosuppressant agent quite similar to FK-506?

A. Azathioprine
B. Cyclosporine
C. Sirolimus
D. Fludrocortisone

MODULE 2 ANSWERS

CASE 1

1a. (E) Asthma is a chronic inflammatory disorder of the airways accompanied by airway hyperresponsiveness and obstruction.

1b. (A) Airway inflammation is recognized as the central component of asthma.

1c. (E) Several airway resident and immigrating cells contribute to the pathophysiology of asthma. Eosinophils and mast cells are the principal inciting cells whereas T-lymphocytes, macrophages, and neutrophils are also involved. These cells are involved either directly or indirectly in the release of inflammatory mediators including histamine, leukotrienes, cytokines, platelet-activating and chemotactic factors, and prostaglandins.

1d. (E) Coughing and breathlessness, especially if at night, after exertion, or after breathing cold air, are indicative of asthma. Wheezing, often accompanied by chest tightness, is also a common sign of asthma.

1e. (A) The respective brand and generic names are: Ventolin and Proventil (albuterol), Vancenase and Vanceril (beclomethasone), and Flovent (fluticasone).

1f. (B) Albuterol administration may result in an apparent hypokalemia because of an intracellular shift of potassium.

1g. (B) During an asthma exacerbation, three doses of albuterol may be administered during the first hour with subsequent dosing based on patient response.

1h. (C) The respective brand and generic names are: Proventil (albuterol), Serevent (salmeterol), Atrovent (ipratropium bromide), and Flovent (fluticasone).

1i. (D) Ipratropium bromide is a synthetic quaternary anticholinergic ammonium compound chemically similar to atropine. When inhaled, it acts locally and is not readily absorbed into the systemic circulation.

1j. (B) The respective brand and generic names are: Vancenase (beclomethasone), Flovent (fluticasone), Serevent (salmeterol), and Azmacort (triamcinolone).

1k. (B)

1l. (C) Fluticasone is a corticosteroid administered via inhalation with an appropriate initial dose of two puffs twice a day. However, during an asthma exacerbation, patients should receive systemic corticosteroids in lieu of the inhaled route. Therefore, an alternative would be to discontinue fluticasone and initiate methylprednisolone 1–2 mg/kg intravenously every 6 hours.

CASE 2

2a. (B) As a result of their rapid onset of action, a β-2 agonist, such as albuterol, is the drug of choice for the initial treatment of status asthmaticus.

2b. (D) The respective brand and generic names are: Solu-Cortef (hydrocortisone), Celestone (betamethasone), Pediapred (prednisolone), and Solu-Medrol (methylprednisolone).

2c. (B)

2d. (B) The initial dose of methylprednisolone for the treatment of status asthmaticus is commonly 1–2 mg/kg. In this case, a 10-fold dosing error occurred as Ali, weighing 25 kg (2.2 lbs/1 kg = 55 lbs/x; x = 25 kg), should have been prescribed 25 mg iv q 6 hours.

2e. (B) Ali is prescribed 2.5 mg per dose. Using the stock solution, 20 mg/1 mL = 2.5 mg/x; x = 0.125 mL or ~ 0.13 mL.

2f. (D) Methylprednisolone is a systemic corticosteroid with several potential adverse effects including hypertension, hyperglycemia, adrenal suppression, pancreatitis, psychosis, edema, hypokalemia, impaired wound healing, immunosuppression, cataracts, glaucoma, impaired growth, osteoporosis, and leukocytosis.

2g. (B) Azithromycin, clarithromycin, and erythromycin are representative of the macrolide class of antibiotics. Ciprofloxacin is a fluoroquinolone, aztreonam is a monobactam, and ticarcillin is a penicillin.

2h. (C) Unlike azithromycin, the macrolides erythromycin and clarithromycin are significant inhibitors of the cytochrome P450 isoenzyme system resulting in several potential drug-drug interactions including decreased clearance of theophylline. Azithromycin does not appear to significantly influence this system, thereby being associated with few drug interactions.

2i. (C) The correct dose of intravenous azithromycin is 10 mg/kg qd (maximum dose = 500 mg). Therefore, Ali (25 kg) should receive 250 mg iv qd (10 mg/kg × 25 kg = 250 mg).

2j. (D) Although the macrolides (i.e., azithromycin) have some activity against gram- positive and gram-negative bacteria, it is most likely prescribed here for its activity against atypical bacteria such as *Mycoplasma*. Also, azithromycin does not possess activity against *Pseudomonas* and it is unlikely that Ali is infected with *Staphylococcus*.

2k. (C)

2l. (A) Elixophyllin, Slo-bid, and Theodur are brand names for theophylline.

2m. (C) The correct loading dose of aminophylline is 6 mg/kg. Therefore, for Ali, 6 mg/kg × 25 kg = 150 mg.

2n. (C) A reasonable initial aminophylline infusion for Ali, a 6 year old, would be 1 mg/kg/hr. Therefore, 1 mg/kg/hr × 25 kg = 25 mg/hr.

2o. (B) Although some patients may benefit from higher concentrations, a theophylline serum concentration of 5–15 mg/L is therapeutic for most. Also, concentrations exceeding 15 mg/L are more likely to result in drug-induced adverse effects.

2p. (C) Steady-state drug concentrations are achieved within 4–5 half-lives of the drug in question regardless of whether a loading dose is prescribed. However, a loading dose does allow for such a dose to be given to result in rapid achievement of a desired drug concentration.

CASE 3

3a. (C) In the treatment of asthma, magnesium is believed to act at the cellular level to antagonize the translocation of calcium across cell membranes including those associated with bronchial smooth muscle. Magnesium may also inhibit the degranulation of mast cells and decrease the amount of acetylcholine released at motor nerve terminals.

3b. (E) Although quite safe, potential adverse effects from magnesium therapy include hypotension, muscle weakness, and respiratory and central nervous system depression. Generally, the more severe adverse effects occur at magnesium concentrations exceeding 7 mg/dL.

3c. (B) Although there is little data and thus no established therapeutic serum concentration range for magnesium for the treatment of asthma, authors have reported concentrations of 4–5 mg/dL to be efficacious and well tolerated.

3d. (B) Although there are no established dosing guidelines for intravenous magnesium in the treatment of asthma, in the presence of normal renal function, a reasonable approach is to prescribe a loading dose of 50 mg/kg (maximum dose = 2 grams) followed by 20–25 mg/kg/hr. For Andre, a loading dose of 50 mg/kg calculates to 3 grams (50 mg/kg × 60 kg = 3000 mg or 3 grams) so he should receive the maximum recommended loading dose of 2 grams followed by ~ 1200 mg/hr (20 mg/kg/hr × 60 kg = 1200 mg/hr). Subsequent dosing should be based on clinical response and observed magnesium serum concentrations. In lieu of a continuous infusion, some have elected to prescribe multiple bolus injections with a range of doses being prescribed.

3e. (D) Andre's loading dose of 25 mg/kg × 60 kg = 1500 mg. Therefore, 80 mg/2 mL = 1500 mg/x; x = 37.5 mL.

3f. (B) Andre's aminophylline dose of 0.7 mg/kg/hr × 60 kg = 42 mg/hr. Hence, 500 mg/500 mL = 42 mg/x; x = 42 mL. Therefore, the rate should be 42 mL/hr.

3g. (D) Intravenous ranitidine is most commonly prescribed as 2–4 mg/kg/day divided every 8 hours with a maximum single dose of 50 mg as the most commonly prescribed dose. Therefore, Andre should be prescribed 50 mg iv q 8 hours (150 mg/day/60 kg = 2.5 mg/kg/day).

3h. (C) Respiratory failure and coagulopathy are the most significant risk factors for the occurrence of stress ulcers. Histamine-2 antagonists (i.e., ranitidine), proton pump inhibitors, or sucralfate are most commonly prescribed for stress ulcer prophylaxis.

3i. (A) Like ranitidine, famotidine (Pepcid) is a histamine-2 antagonist.

3j. (A) Omeprazole, a proton pump inhibitor, is also prescribed for stress ulcer prophylaxis.

CASE 4

4a. (A) For the treatment of asthma, ketamine is typically dosed at a 0.5–1.0 mg/kg loading dose followed by 0.5–1.0 mg/kg/hr. Therefore, David might receive 0.5 mg/kg followed by 40 mg/hr (1 mg/kg/hr × 40 kg = 40 mg/hr).

4b. (A) The mechanism of ketamine's bronchodilating activity appears to be an increase in synaptic catecholamine concentrations as well as inhibiting vagal outflow.

4c. (E) Ketamine's adverse effects include increased oral and tracheal secretions, cardiovascular stimulation, increased intraocular and intracranial pressure, and emergent reactions including hallucinations, nightmares, and delirium.

4d. (A) Anticholinergics, such as atropine, are often prescribed to decrease the secretions resulting from ketamine therapy. Benzodiazepines are also prescribed to reduce the risk of the emergent reactions. David is already receiving a benzodiazepine (lorazepam) and, therefore, diazepam (Valium), also a benzodiazepine, should not be prescribed.

4e. (B) The respective brand and generic names are: Biaxin (clarithromycin), Zithromax (azithromycin), Azactam (aztreonam), E-mycin (erythromycin).

4f. (C) Although erythromycin and clarithromycin have similar antimicrobial activity as azithromycin, a drug-drug interaction between erythromycin or clarithromycin and aminophylline would have the potential to result in toxic theophylline concentrations. Therefore, the macrolide of choice for David would be azithromycin. The correct intravenous dose for David is 400 mg (10 mg/kg × 40 kg = 400 mg) iv qd. It is available in both oral and intravenous dosage forms.

4g. (D) Lorazepam (Ativan) is a benzodiazepine.

4h. (D) A reasonable initial dose of intravenous lorazepam would be 0.05–0.1 mg/kg/hr.

4i. (D) For David, 0.15 mg/kg/hr × 40 kg = 6 mg/hr × 24 hours = 144 mg.

4j. (B) Adverse effects of neuromuscular-blocking agents include prolonged paralysis and myopathy. Coadministration of corticosteroids (i.e., methylprednisolone) or aminoglycosides (i.e., gentamicin) is known to increase the risk of such adverse effects.

4k. (B) Intravenous ranitidine is most commonly prescribed as 2–4 mg/kg/day divided every 8 hours.

4l. (C) David's ranitidine dose is 40 mg. Using a 25 mg/mL solution; 25 mg/1 mL = 40 mg/x; x = 1.6 mL.

4m. (D) Although there are few data and thus no established therapeutic serum concentration range for magnesium for the treatment of asthma, authors have reported concentrations of 4–5 mg/dL to be efficacious and well tolerated. With a reported concentration of 4.1 mg/dL in David and in the absence of adverse effects, the dosage should be maintained.

4n. (C) Although rare, β-2 agonists (i.e., albuterol) have the potential to result in increased lactate concentrations indicative of metabolic acidosis.

4o. (C) Aminophylline is 80% theophylline. Therefore 6 mg/kg of aminophylline = 4.8 mg/kg theophylline (0.8 × 6 = 4.8). Using the equation: Concentration = Dose/Volume of Distribution; Concentration = 4.8 mg/kg/0.5 L/kg = 9.6 mg/L.

CASE 5

5a. (D) Status epilepticus is a common true emergency among pediatric patients and is defined as continuous seizure activity for longer than 30 minutes or the occurrence of two or more seizures without full recovery of consciousness during the interictal period.

5b. (E) Examples of seizure precipitants include trauma, infections, fever, metabolic disturbances, congenital defects, anoxia, strokes, tumors, alcohol, or medications. For approximately 25% of the cases, the etiology of the seizure is not defined.

5c. (D) During the early stages of a seizure, enhanced autonomic activity manifest as tachycardia, hypertension, hyperglycemia, and hyperthermia.

5d. (C) Although both lorazepam and diazepam are benzodiazepines and are both highly effective in the treatment of status epilepticus, lorazepam typically exhibits a longer duration of initial seizure control, and is therefore the preferred drug by most clinicians.

5e. (D) Lorazepam is less lipid soluble than diazepam and thus has a slightly delayed onset of action compared with diazepam. However, its effects are noticed within minutes and its duration of action for seizure control is longer than that of diazepam.

5f. (C) Fosphenytoin is a prodrug of phenytoin that is rapidly converted to phenytoin by endogenous phosphatases. Compared with phenytoin, it is more water soluble, does not contain propylene glycol, and may be administered intramuscularly. However, it is substantially more expensive than phenytoin.

5g. (B) The recommended loading dose of fosphenytoin is 15–20 mg/kg PE with the infusion rate not to exceed 3 mg PE/kg/min or 150 min.

5h. (A) Fosphenytoin is dosed based on phenytoin sodium equivalents. The conversion is 75 mg of fosphenytoin = 50 mg phenytoin.

5i. (C) It is recommended to obtain a phenytoin peak concentration no sooner than 2 hours after a fosphenytoin dose.

5j. (B) Since fosphenytoin is dosed in phenytoin sodium equivalents, the same dose of phenytoin would be prescribed.

5k. (D) When treating status epilepticus, a phenytoin peak concentration of ~ 25 mg/L (mcg/mL) is often targeted. The therapeutic range for phenytoin trough concentrations during maintenance therapy is 10–20 mcg/mL.

5l. (B) The respective brand and generic names are: Celebrex (celecoxib), Cerebyx (fosphenytoin), Cefadyl (cephapirin), and Cedax (ceftibuten).

5m. (A) For Donte, lorazepam should be prescribed at 0.05–0.1 mg/kg.

5n. (D) The dose of lorazepam for status epilepticus is 0.05–0.1 mg/kg with a recommended maximum single dose of 4 mg. Since Donte is 40 kg, he could receive the maximum recommended single dose of 4 mg (0.1 mg/kg × 40 kg = 4 mg).

CASE 6

6a. (A) The maximum recommended infusion rate for phenytoin is 1 mg/kg/min, not to exceed 50 mg/min.

6b. (C) Initial dosing of phenytoin usually includes a loading dose of 15–20 mg/kg followed by 5 mg/kg/day divided every 12 hours.

6c. (D) Jenny's phenytoin concentration is slightly below the recommended therapeutic range of 10–20 mcg/mL. With continued seizure activity, it is prudent to target a higher concentration than her current value of 9 mcg/mL. A loading dose of 10 mg/kg would increase her to approximately 24 mcg/mL (Concentration = Dose/Volume of distribution; Volume of distribution = ~ 0.7 L/kg. Therefore, a dose of 10 mg/kg would increase the concentration by ~ 14 mg/L; Concentration = 10 mg/kg/ 0.7 L/kg = 15 mg/L; 15 mg/L + her current value of 9 mg/L = 24 mg/L). It would also be necessary to increase her maintenance dose to prevent her phenytoin concentration from eventually returning to her prebolus concentration. A reasonable initial regimen would be 5 mg/kg/day divided every 12 hours.

6d. (B) Concentration = Dose/Volume of distribution. To convert her dose to dose/kg; 200 mg/27 kg = 7.4 mg/kg. Therefore, Concentration = 7.4 mg/kg / 0.7 L/kg = 10.6 mg/L. Hence, a phenytoin dose of 200 mg would raise her concentration by ~ 11 mg/L that when added to her current serum concentration of 9 mg/L would result in a serum concentration of 20 mg/L (11 mg/L + 9 mg/L = 20 mg/L).

6e. (C)

6f. (D) A reasonable initial pediatric phenobarbital regimen is 5 mg/kg/day divided every 12 hours.

Therapy is most often initiated with a loading dose of 15–20 mg/kg.

6g. (D) The recommended phenobarbital loading dose is 15–20 mg/kg. For Jenny, 27 kg × 20 mg/kg = 540 mg = ~ 550 mg.

6h. (C)

6i. (D) Midazolam is a water soluble benzodiazepine and has a very short elimination half-life ranging from ~ 1–3 hours. It has proven successful in the treatment of refractory status epilepticus.

6j. (D) For the treatment of seizures, midazolam may be initiated at a loading dose of 0.15 mg/kg followed by an infusion of 1 mcg/kg/min. For refractory seizures, the midazolam infusion has been titrated up to 24 mcg/kg/min.

6k. (B) The respective brand and generic names are: Valium (diazepam), Versed (midazolam), Vasotec (enalapril), and Ventolin (albuterol).

6l. (C) Both midazolam and diazepam are benzodiazepines.

6m. (E)

6n. (B) Midazolam therapy should be weaned off to potentially prevent withdrawal or recurrence of seizure. If seizure activity occurs during the weaning, it would be prudent to resume at the previous dose at which no seizure activity occurred. Once the patient is stable, the weaning may once again be resumed. A reasonable midazolam wean would be by 1–2 mcg/kg/min every 15 minutes until discontinued.

CASE 7

7a. (B)

7b. (B) An appropriate loading dose of pentobarbital is 10–15 mg/kg infused over 1–2 hours. Therefore, for Sam, 35 kg × 10 mg/kg = 350 mg.

7c. (D) Therapeutic serum concentrations of pentobarbital for sedation, hypnosis, and coma are 1–5 mg/L, 5–15 mg/L, and 20–40 mg/L, respectively. Therefore, a targeted serum concentration of 20–40 mg/L would be reasonable for Sam.

7d. (B) Sam's daily dose is 70 mg/hr × 24 hours = 1680 mg. Therefore, using a 50 mg/mL solution; 50 mg/mL = 1680 mg/x; x = 33.6 mL.

7e. (B) The respective brand and generic names are: Seconal (secobarbital), Nembutal (pentobarbital), Mebaral (mephobarbital), and Solfoton (phenobarbital).

7f. (B) The respective brand and generic names are: Ditropan (oxybutynin), Diprivan (propofol), Demadex (torsemide), and Dalmane (flurazepam).

7g. (B) Sam's daily propofol dose is 3 mg/kg/hr × 35 kg × 24 h = 2520 mg. Therefore, he will receive 252 mLs of propofol per day (10 mg/mL = 2520 mg/x; x = 252 mLs. A 10% intralipid base contains 10 grams/100 mL. Hence, 10 grams/100 mL = x/252 mL; x = 25.2 grams of intralipid per day.

7h. (C) Because propofol is a 10% intravenous fat emulsion, serum triglycerides should be monitored closely during therapy. Additionally, a patient receiving intravenous lipids who is prescribed propofol should have the intravenous fat dose adjusted to account for the amount of lipids that will be received via the propofol dose.

7i. (E) Propofol's sedative effects usually dissipate within 30 minutes of drug discontinuation. Administration may result in hypotension or apnea especially following bolus doses or in patients who are hypovolemic. Due to potential contamination, the drug and iv tubing should be replaced every 12 hours.

7j. (C) Propofol lowers intracranial pressure. It is associated with constriction of cerebral arteries and decreased cerebral blood flow accompanied by reduced cerebral metabolic requirements.

7k. (A) The maximum recommended infusion rate for phenytoin is 1 mg/kg/min not to exceed 50 mg/min. With Sam being 35 kg, his maximum recommended rate would be 35 mg/min (1 mg/kg/min × 35 kg = 35 mg/min).

7l. (B) Sam's daily dose is 180 mg (90 mg q 12 h). The stock solution is 50 mg/mL. Therefore, 50 mg/mL = 180 mg/x; x = 3.6 mL.

CASE 8

8a. (E) Clinical signs of elevated intracranial pressure include papilledema, bradycardia, bradypnea, fixed pupils unresponsive to light, flaccidity, posturing, vomiting, and hypertension. Symptoms include headache, diplopia, decreased vision, and slow mentation.

8b. (D) Normal intracranial pressure is considered to be less than 15 mm Hg.

8c. (B) Cerebral perfusion pressure (CPP) = mean arterial pressure (MAP) – intracranial pressure (ICP); MAP = 2/3 diastolic blood pressure + 1/3 systolic blood pressure. For Cary (B/P = 120/60),

MAP = (2/3 × 60) + (1/3 × 120) = 80. Hence, CPP = 80 − 22 = 58 mm Hg.

8d. (A) Cerebral blood flow is markedly decreased when cerebral perfusion pressure falls below 50 mm Hg and virtually ceases with values below 20 mm Hg.

8e. (E)

8f. (B)

8g. (A) Serum osmolality should be routinely monitored during mannitol therapy with the dose being administered only when the serum osmolality is below 320 mOsm/L. Mannitol 20% has an approximate osmolality of 1100 mOsm/L.

8h. (B) Serum osmolality is calculated as: 2 × serum sodium + serum glucose/18 + BUN/2.8. Therefore, for Cary, the calculated serum osmolality is (2 × 135) + (150/18) + (7/2.8) = 281 mOsm/L.

8i. (D) Severe adverse effects are more common when the serum osmolality exceeds 320 mOsm/L. Therefore, mannitol dosing is usually withheld when the serum osmolality exceeds such value.

8j. (B) As a result of mannitol's rapid renal clearance, its duration of action is approximately 4 hours.

8k. (D) Maintenance dosing of mannitol is usually 0.25–0.5 gm/kg every 4 to 6 hours. Therefore, a reasonable dose for Cary would be 10 grams (0.25 gms × 40 kg) every 4 hours. Subsequent dosing should be based on response and serum osmolality.

8l. (E) Other therapies to lower intracranial pressure include hypertonic saline solutions, propofol, pentobarbital, loop diuretics, and in some cases corticosteroids.

8m. (D) Hyperventilation results in a decrease in arterial carbon dioxide tension (PCO$_2$) to ~ 25–30 mm Hg. The lower PCO$_2$ results in cerebral vasoconstriction that leads to a reduction in cerebral blood volume and a decrease in intracranial pressure. Upon discontinuation of hyperventilation, the PCO$_2$ must be allowed to return slowly to normal to avoid a rebound elevation in intracranial pressure.

8n. (C) Loading doses of pentobarbital for the treatment of elevated intracranial pressure normally range from 3–10 mg/kg with maintenance doses ranging from 1–3 mg/kg/hr. Therefore, for Cary, a 400 mg loading dose (40 kg × 10 mg/kg) followed by 1 mg/kg/hr would be a more reasonable regimen.

8o. (A) Several mechanisms have been postulated in reference to the benefits of pentobarbital for the treatment of increased intracranial pressure (ICP). It may lower ICP by increasing cerebrovascular resistance thereby decreasing cerebral blood flow and volume. It may also decrease the energy requirements of the brain in the presence of hypoxia thereby maintaining cerebral function. Vasoconstriction of cerebral vessels also occurs, which results in blood being shunted from normal to ischemic areas. Cerebral vasoconstriction may also reduce edema formation resulting in decreased ICP. Finally, it may act as a scavenger of free oxygen radicals that may cause cellular brain damage.

CASE 9

9a. (E)

9b. (D) Alka-Seltzer Plus Cold and Cough Tablets contain aspirin in lieu of acetaminophen.

9c. (B) Toxic doses of acetaminophen saturate the glucuronic and sulfate metabolic pathways resulting in excessive amounts being metabolized through the cytochrome P-450 isoenzyme system to a toxic metabolite, N-acetylimidoquinone. This toxic metabolite appears to be responsible for the acetaminophen-induced hepatotoxicity.

9d. (D)

9e. (E) Prothrombin time (PT) and liver function tests (ALT, AST, GGT) are often obtained to assist in determining the degree of toxicity from acetaminophen.

9f. (A) Following a significant ingestion of acetaminophen, compared with AST and ALT values, a change in prothrombin time is often manifested more acutely.

9g. (B)

9h. (C) Extra strength acetaminophen capsules contain 500 mg/capsule. Therefore, 50 capsules (the number ingested by Melissa) $\times$ 500 mg = 25,000 mg; 25,000 mg/63 kg = 397 mg/kg or $\sim$ 400 mg/kg.

9i. (B)

9j. (C) Her dose of 50 mg/kg $\times$ 63 kg = 3150 mg or 3.15 gms. A 20% solution of Mucomyst = 20 gms/100 mLs. Therefore, 20 gms/100 mLs = 3.15 gms/x; x = 15.75 mLs.

9k. (C) The proper loading dose of Mucomyst is 140 mg/kg. Therefore, 140 mg/kg $\times$ 63 kg = 8820 mg or $\sim$ 8800 mg.

9l. (C) Mucomyst acts as an antidote for acetaminophen toxicity by providing a glutathione substitute in the face of glutathione depletion to detoxify the reactive metabolite, N-acetylimidoquinone, and to enhance the sulfation of acetaminophen. Mucomyst is most effective when administered within 8–12 hours of the acetaminophen ingestion.

9m. (B) The value of the acetaminophen concentration obtained at least 4 hours postingestion should be plotted on the Rumack nomogram to assess the degree of toxicity and the need for Mucomyst therapy. The plotted value will indicate either probable, possible, or no hepatic toxicity.

9n. (B) Four hours following the Mucomyst oral loading dose of 140 mg/kg, Melissa should receive 70 mg/kg orally every 4 hours for 17 additional doses.

9o. (A) Activated charcoal does not appear to alter the disposition of Mucomyst, and therefore dosage adjustments are not necessary.

9p. (B) The respective trade and generic names are: Lotronex (alosetron), Zofran (ondansetron), Kytril (granisetron), and Anzemet (dolasetron).

9q. (B) Because of the "sulfur" component of Mucomyst, nausea and vomiting are common adverse effects that can usually be controlled with ondansetron or metoclopramide.

9r. (C)

CASE 10

10a. (A) The respective trade and generic names are: Tegretol (carbamazepine), Tenormin (atenolol), Trental (pentoxifylline), and Timoptic (timolol).

10b. (D)

10c. (E) The therapeutic anticonvulsant activity of carbamazepine is primarily the blockade of presynaptic voltage-dependent sodium channels. It also inhibits muscarinic and nicotinic acetylcholine receptors, N-methyl-D-aspartate receptors, and central nervous system adenosine receptors. It also may affect cardiac sodium channels.

10d. (B)

10e. (E) The toxicity profile of carbamazepine mostly involves neurologic and cardiac manifestations including coma, respiratory depression, seizures, and ventricular arrhythmias.

10f. (B)

10g. (A) In overdose, absorption of carbamazepine is often slow and erratic; peak concentrations are delayed up to 70 hours postdose. It also has substantial anticholinergic effects that may produce ileus. At therapeutic doses, carbamazepine only has minimal effects on the cardiac sodium channels; however, at higher doses, it may be proarrhythmic.

10h. (A) The benzodiazepines (i.e., lorazepam) are the preferred drugs for the treatment of carbamazepines induced seizures. Phenytoin shares a similar mechanism of action with carbamazepine (i.e., blockade of sodium channels) and, therefore, is not recommended. Carbatrol is a longer-acting carbamazepine preparation.

10i. (A) Repeat doses of activated charcoal are often prescribed between 0.25–1 gm/kg. Therefore, 500 mg/kg (0.5 gm/kg) would be an appropriate dose for Courtney.

10j. (B) Multiple dose activated charcoal has been proven effective in enhancing clearance of excessive doses of carbamazepine. However, carbamazepine's anticholinergic property does warrant careful monitoring of bowel function to ensure adequate elimination. Initial doses of activated charcoal may be administered in a sorbitol base to enhance elimination; however, continued use of sorbitol during multiple dosing is not recommended.

10k. (C) Activated charcoal should not be mixed with milk or ice cream and rapid consumption may increase the risk of vomiting. A minimum dilution of 240 mLs per 20–30 grams is recommended. Charcoal turns the stools black in color. Caution should be exercised in obtunded patients as aspiration may lead to tracheal obstruction.

10l. (D) A dose of 10,000 mgs = 10 gms. Therefore, 25 gms/120 mLs = 10 gms/x; x = 48 or ~ 50 mLs.

CASE 11

11a. (D) Normal magnesium serum concentration ranges from 1.6–2.4 mEq/L. Therefore, it would be reasonable to provide John with a 25–50 mg/kg intravenous dose of magnesium sulfate to correct his low concentration of 1.4 mEq/L. A subsequent magnesium concentration should be obtained and further supplements provided if needed.

11b. (E) In the presence of a bacterial infection, total white blood cell count (WBC) and immature white cells (bands) are often increased. C-reactive protein (CRP), an acute phase reactant, is also often elevated in the presence of a bacterial infectious process.

11c. (D) Zosyn is a combination product containing piperacillin and tazobactam. Piperacillin is an extended spectrum penicillin while tazobactam is a β-lactamase inhibitor.

11d. (E) Zosyn is an extended spectrum penicillin that provides antibacterial coverage against a range of bacteria including *Pseudomonas*, a gram-negative aerobic bacteria.

11e. (A) Timentin is also classified as an extended spectrum penicillin as is Zosyn, and provides similar antibacterial coverage.

11f. (D) The correct dose of dopamine for John would be 15 mcg/kg/min. Normal dosing range is 1–20 mcg/kg/min. Initially, fentanyl is typically dosed at 1–3 mcg/kg/hr, vancomycin at 15–20 mg/kg, and lorazepam at 0.05–0.1 mg/kg/hr.

11g. (B) The half-life is the time required for a concentration to decrease by one half. Therefore, a decrease from 28 mcg/mL to 7 mcg/mL represents 2 half-lives (i.e., decreased by one half twice; 28 to 14 to 7). Since this occurred over a 6-hour period (from 1300 to 1900), the 6 hours represents two half-lives or 3 hours per half-life. Half-life can also be calculated by the equation: Half-life = $0.693/k_e$, where 0.693 is a constant and k_e is the elimination rate constant. The k_e is calculated as $k_e = \ln (C_{peak}/C_{trough})/\Delta time$. In this example, $k_e = \ln (28/7)/6$ hours = 0.231/hr; half-life = 0.693/0.231 = 2.99 hours or 3 hours.

11h. (D) The effects of dopamine are dose dependent. In general, at low doses (~1–5 mcg/kg/min), dopaminergic receptors are predominately affected. At intermediate doses (~ 5–15 mcg/kg/min) β-receptors are affected with α-receptors being predominately affected at doses > 15 mcg/kg/min.

11i. (A)

11j. (B) Dopamine is rapidly metabolized by monoamine oxidase and catechol-o-methyltransferase resulting in a half-life of ~ 2 minutes. Therefore, to maintain adequate concentrations and effects, dopamine is administered via continuous infusion.

11k. (C) The respective trade and generic names are: Dobutrex (dobutamine), Inocor (amrinone), Intropin (dopamine), and Primacor (milrinone).

11l. (B) Phentolamine is an α-adrenergic antagonist used as local treatment of tissue necrosis from extravasation of drugs with α-adrenergic effects (i.e., dopamine, dobutamine, epinephrine, norepinephrine, and phenylephrine).

11m. (C) The proper initial pediatric dose of tobramycin is 2.5 mg/kg/dose iv q 8 hours. Therefore, John should receive ~ 38 mg (2.5 mg/kg × 15 kg) with subsequent dosing based on pharmacokinetic analysis from concentrations obtained.

11n. (B) For John, tobramycin was likely prescribed to provide additional coverage for *Pseudomonas*, a gram-negative bacteria. To prevent resistance and promote additional bactericidal activity against *Pseudomonas*, many clinicians prefer to provide double anti-pseudomonal coverage.

11o. (B) High serum-peak concentrations (i.e., 8–10 or 8–12 mcg/mL) of tobramycin are recommended for pulmonary infections. To reduce the risk of toxicity, trough concentrations below 2 mcg/mL are recommended.

11p. (B) By convention, third-dose peak and trough concentrations are often requested by which time it is assumed tobramycin steady-state conditions have been attained. However, by altering pharmacokinetic equations, a pharmacokinetic analysis may be performed on alternate doses as well.

CASE 12

12a. (B) The respective trade and generic names are: Adrenalin (epinephrine), Levophed (norepinephrine), Primacor (milrinone), and Nitropress (nitroprusside).

12b. (A) Norepinephrine stimulates α- and β-receptors. Stimulation of α-1 receptors results in vasoconstriction. Clinically, the alpha-effects (vasoconstriction) are greater than the beta-effects (inotropic and chronotropic).

12c. (E) Because of its multiple benefits, norepinephrine is the preferred vasopressor by many clinicians for the treatment of septic shock. Its benefits include: attenuation of inappropriate vasodilatation and low-oxygen extraction, attenuation of myocardial depression, improvement of renal perfusion and filtration, and improvement of splanchnic perfusion.

12d. (E) Potential adverse effects of norepinephrine include hypertension, photophobia, chest pain, intense sweating, cerebral hemorrhaging, seizures, arrhythmias, bradycardia, tachycardia, and anxiety.

12e. (A) The usual dosage range for norepinephrine is 0.05–2 mcg/kg/min. Therefore, Seth should have been prescribed 0.08 mcg/kg/min instead of 0.008 mcg/kg/min, representing a 10-fold dosing error.

12f. (B) In the event vasopressor agents fail to improve a patient's blood pressure, it would be reasonable to access the patient's adrenal function by obtaining a

cortisol concentration and/or performing an adrenal stimulation test.

12g. (B) Aminoglycosides (i.e., gentamicin) have been shown to increase the risks of adverse effects (prolonged paralysis, myopathy) from neuromuscular blocking agents.

12h. (B) Train of four (peripheral nerve stimulation) is a technique that delivers a series of electrical stimuli through electrodes applied to the skin over a peripheral nerve. In this case, the ulnar nerve is given four small electrical stimuli consecutively every half second to elicit contraction of the thumb adductor muscle. The number of "thumb twitches" out of four stimulations defines the degree of neuromuscular blockade: 0/4 = 100% blockade, 1/4 = 90% blockade, 2/4 = 75 % blockade, 3/4 =<50% blockade, 4/4 = 0% blockade. Ideally, 1/4 or 2/4 twitches is desired for optimal neuromuscular blockade.

12i. (D) Vecuronium is a derivative of pancuronium, a long-acting neuromuscular blocker. Unlike pancuronium, vecuronium does not cause catecholamine or histamine release.

12j. (D) Cisatracurium (Nimbex) is metabolized via spontaneous degradation at physiologic pH and temperature (Hofmann elimination) and therefore does not depend on renal or hepatic function for elimination.

12k. (B) Timentin contains an extended spectrum penicillin (ticarcillin) and a β-lactamase inhibitor (clavulanate).

12l. (B) Timentin and ceftazidime have a similar spectrum of activity against microbes including activity against *Pseudomonas*. Unlike ceftazidime, Timentin provides coverage against anaerobes.

12m. (C) Depakote and Depakene are oral formulations of valproic acid. Dilantin is a brand name for phenytoin.

12n. (D) Although 50–100 mcg/mL is the therapeutic range of valproic acid for most patients, some require concentrations up to 150 mcg/mL for control of seizure activity.

12o. (A) Given Seth's "normal" sodium concentration and "low" potassium concentration, it would be more appropriate to replenish his serum phosphate with potassium phosphate. Injectable potassium phosphate contains 4.4 mEq of potassium and 3 mMol of phosphorus per milliliter.

12p. (C) Seth's sodium phosphate order implies 0.2 mMol of phosphorus per kg. Therefore, 0.2 mMol ×

19 kg = 3.8 mMol of phosphorus. Sodium phosphate contains 3 mMol of phosphorus and 4 mEq of sodium per milliliter. So, 3 mMol phosphorus/4 mEq sodium = 3.8 mMol phosphorus/x; x = 5.1 mEq sodium.

12q. (C) Because of its low renal threshold, sodium or potassium phosphate should be infused over a minimum of 4–6 hours.

12r. (B) Valproic acid therapy may result in hyperammonemia, with or without coma, in the absence of abnormal liver function tests. The drug may increase renal ammonia production and inhibit urea synthesis. Therefore, patients should be monitored for potential hepatotoxicity.

12s. (B) Lactulose enhances the diffusion of NH_3 from the blood into the gut where the conversion to NH_4 occurs. Neomycin, an aminoglycoside antibiotic, is also used in the treatment of hyperammonemia.

12t. (C) Calcium gluconate 10% = 10 gms/100 mL. Therefore, 10 gms/100 mL = 1.9 gms/x; x = 19 mLs.

12u. (B) One gram of calcium gluconate = 4.5 mEq of elemental calcium. Therefore, 1 gm calcium gluconate/4.5 mEq calcium = 1.9 gm calcium gluconate/x; x = 8.6 mEq elemental calcium.

CASE 13

13a. (E) Presenting signs and symptoms of meningitis include fever, headache, neck stiffness, nausea, vomiting, photophobia, lethargy, and irritability.

13b. (B) Kernig's sign is flexion of the hip 90 degrees with subsequent pain with extension of the leg.

13c. (A) Normally, CSF is clear with a protein content < 50 mg/dL, a glucose concentration of 50–66% of the serum glucose, a pH of 7.4, and fewer than 5 WBCs per mm^3.

13d. (E) Typically with bacterial meningitis, the CSF protein is between 100–500 mg/dL, the CSF glucose is < 40 mg/dL, and the CSF polymorphonuclear cells (PMNs) > 75%.

13e. (D)

13f. (A) Previously, *Haemophilus influenzae* was the most common pathogen associated with meningitis. However, subsequent to the *H. influenzae* vaccine, *Streptococcus pneumoniae* has become the most common cause of meningitis.

13g. (A) The respective brand and generic names are: Claforan (cefotaxime), Ceftin (cefuroxime), Mefoxin (cefoxitin), and Rocephin (ceftriaxone).

13h. (C)

13i. (C) The recommended cefotaxime dose for meningitis is 300 mg/kg/day divided every 6 hours. Therefore, William should receive 300 mg/kg/day × 11 kg = 3300 mg/day or ~ 800 mg every 6 hours.

13j. (B) Ceftriaxone (Rocephin) is another third generation cephalosporin indicated for the empiric treatment of meningitis. The meningitic ceftriaxone dose is 100 mg/kg/day given either once or twice daily not to exceed 2 grams per dose.

13k. (A) With the emergence of resistant strains of *Streptococcus pneumoniae*, vancomycin in a dose of 60 mg/kg/day is recommended to be combined with a third-generation cephalosporin in the treatment of infants and children with suspected meningitis.

13l. (D) Dexamethasone, when administered before antibiotics, modulates the enhanced meningeal inflammatory response because of transcriptional events for tumor necrosis factor and interleukin-1 production being inhibited. Also, dexamethasone has been shown to lessen hearing loss, the most frequent sequelae associated with meningeal inflammation, in patients with *H. influenzae* type b meningitis.

13m. (C) The correct dose of dexamethasone as adjunct therapy for meningitis is 0.15 mg/kg iv q 6 hours. Therefore, 0.15 mg/kg × 11 kg = 1.7 mg.

13n. (A) Following antibiotic administration, rapid bacterial cell lysis results in the release of bacterial cell wall and membrane fragments resulting in an augmented inflammatory response. Therefore, to be effective, dexamethasone must be administered prior to or with the first antibiotic dose.

13o. (C) Dexamethasone 1.1 mg × 4 doses per day = 4.4 mg/day. Therefore, 4 mg/mL = 4.4 mg/x; x = 1.1 mL.

13p. (A) Although the data is not supportive of routine use of ranitidine for the prevention of steroid induced gastrointestinal adverse effects, it is likely this was the rationale for prescribing it to William.

CASE 14

14a. (B) Respiratory syncytial virus (RSV) is an enveloped, single-stranded RNA virus. It contains two glycosylated surface proteins, G and F. The G-protein is important for attachment to the cell and the F-protein is responsible for fusing viral particles to target cells and for fusing infected cells to neighboring cells, resulting in the characteristic syncytia formation. RSV isolates are of 2 major groups: A and B, with RSV a infection generally being more severe.

14b. (B) Respiratory syncytial virus spreads easily from person to person through respiratory secretions. The eyes and nose are the primary entry sites. RSV secretions can survive on countertops for more than 6 hours and can be recovered from rubber gloves for 90 minutes, from gowns for 30 minutes, and from hands for 25 minutes. RSV is shed for prolonged periods—up to 21 days, or beyond 6 weeks in immunocompromised patients.

14c. (D) Nearly all children are infected with RSV by 2 years of age.

14d. (E) The most concerning effects of respiratory syncytial virus are respiratory depression or apnea. More commonly, patients present with wheezing, rales, nasal discharge, pharyngitis, fever, and cough.

14e. (E) Risk factors for severe respiratory syncytial virus infection include congenital heart disease, pulmonary hypertension, bronchopulmonary dysplasia, cystic fibrosis, immunodeficiency, prematurity, younger than 6 weeks of age, neurologic or metabolic disease, and major congenital anomalies.

14f. (C) Most clinical studies have found little benefit from aerosols in the treatment of RSV. Of those studied, racemic epinephrine appears to provide the most benefit.

14g. (A) Albuterol and Atrovent solutions for nebulization may be combined and administered at the same time.

14h. (A) The respective trade and generic names are: Vaponefrin (racemic epinephrine), Velban (vinblastine), Vasodilan (isoxsuprine), and Vascor (bepridil).

14i. (B)

14j. (A) The mainstay of treatment for RSV is supportive care. In most studies, corticosteroids have not been proven to be beneficial. Ribavirin is the only drug specifically indicated for the treatment of RSV: however, its benefit regarding duration of mechanical ventilation, supplemental oxygenation, intensive care, or hospitalization has not been demonstrated conclusively.

14k. (A) The respective trade and generic names are: Virazole (ribavirin), Synagis (palivizumab), RespiGam (respiratory syncytial virus immune globulin), and CytoGam (cytomegalovirus immune globulin).

14l. (B) Ribavirin is a virustatic agent and is therefore theoretically more effective when administered early in the course of a RSV infection. Although no such data is available in humans, it is a known teratogen in laboratory animals.

14m. (C) Ribavirin is administered via a small particle aerosol generator, also known as a SPAG-2.

14n. (C) Until recently, ribavirin was administered over 12 to 18 hours as a 20 mg/mL solution. Recently, intermittent dosing with 2 grams over 2 hours three times a day as a 60 mg/mL solution has been used.

14o. (E) The major problems associated with ribavirin center around drug administration including ventilator malfunctioning resulting from precipitated drug in ventilatory tubing. Other potential side effects include rash, bronchospasm, hypotension, or worsening respiratory function.

CASE 15

15a. (E) Acute sickle cell pain is unpredictable and may have no identifiable precipitating factor. However, such episodes may be provoked by temperature extremes, changes in altitude, physical and emotional stress, dehydration, menstruation, fatigue, or infections.

15b. (E) The most common sites of sickle cell pain are the lower back, thigh, hip, knee, abdomen, and chest. For individual patients, pain tends to recur in the same areas and may occur in more than one area at a time.

15c. (A) Sickle cell pain results from tissue ischemia caused by occlusion of vascular beds with sickled erythrocytes.

15d. (A) Most clinicians prefer the use of parenteral opiates for the initial management of acute sickle cell pain.

15e. (B) In the initial management of acute sickle cell pain, patients should be prescribed parenteral opiates at frequent, fixed intervals until the pain has diminished at which time the opiate can be weaned and discontinued with alternative analgesics provided as desired.

15f. (B) The respective trade and generic names are: MS Contin (morphine), Demerol (meperidine), Dilaudid (hydromorphone), and Oxycontin (oxycodone).

15g. (C) Initial intermittent dosing of meperidine to a 44 kg sickle cell patient should be 1–1.5 mg/kg iv every 3–4 hours. Therefore, a reasonable dose would be 50 mg (50 mg/44 kg = 1.1 mg/kg) iv q 4 h.

15h. (B) Normeperidine, an active metabolite of meperidine, is also a central nervous system stimulant that can elicit seizure activity.

15i. (D) Given Tiffany's elevated serum creatinine and thus the possibility of renal impairment, meperidine is not a preferred drug for her as accumulation of its metabolite, normeperidine, may result in seizure activity. A parenteral opiate such as morphine or fentanyl would be reasonable alternatives.

15j. (A) 10 mg of iv morphine is equivalent to 75 mg of iv meperidine. Therefore, 10 mg morphine/x = 75 mg meperidine/25 mg meperidine; x = 3.33 mg morphine or ~ 3.5 mg.

15k. (C) The respective trade and generic names are: Orudis (ketoprofen), Voltaren (diclofenac), Toradol (ketorolac), and Miltown (meprobamate).

15l. (B) Ketorolac is the only available parenteral nonsteroidal anti-inflammatory agent.

15m. (E) As all nonsteroidal anti-inflammatory agents, the adverse effect profile of ketorolac includes renal impairment, gastrointestinal bleeding, and altered platelet function.

15n. (D) The correct pediatric dose of ketorolac is 0.5–1 mg/kg iv q 6 hours, not to exceed 30 mg per dose. However, in the presence of an increased serum creatinine as is present in Tiffany, ketorolac would not be a preferred drug.

15o. (E)

15p. (A) Given its potential adverse effect profile, namely gastrointestinal effects, it is recommended to limit a course of ketorolac therapy to a maximum of 5 days.

CASE 16

16a. (A) Diabetic ketoacidosis (DKA) is characterized by elevated serum glucose, high ketone bodies, and metabolic acidosis. Findings include a serum glucose > 250 mg/dL, an arterial pH < 7.3, and a serum bicarbonate < 15 mEq/L.

16b. (E) Particularly in adolescents, non-compliance with insulin therapy is a major reason of recurrent DKA. Other precipitating events include trauma, febrile illness, psychological stress, and poor sick-day diabetes management.

16c. (B) Cerebral edema occurs in approximately 1% of diabetic ketoacidosis episodes and is associated with a mortality rate of 40 to 90%. It is responsible for ~ 60% of diabetes related deaths in pediatric patients.

16d. (E) Initially, DKA patients often present with normal or elevated serum potassium concentrations that tend to decline as treatment is initiated. Most patients present with an elevated white blood cell count as a stress response, but the count rarely exceeds 25,000/mm³ in the absence of a bacterial infection. Naturally, ketone bodies are present.

16e. (E) An elevated urinary-specific gravity is indicative of dehydration of which is common among DKA patients. The presence of glucose and ketones in the urine is also diagnostic of diabetic ketoacidosis.

16f. (B) Hydration constitutes the most important aspect of the initial management of DKA patients. Hydration provides the necessary fluid to restore intravascular volume and decreases blood concentrations of several counter-regulatory hormones, thus making cells more responsive to insulin therapy.

16g. (A) Isotonic solutions, such as normal saline, are directed toward expansion of extracellular space and more rapidly correct plasma volume than hypotonic solutions. Hypotonic saline is similar to fluid lost during osmotic diuresis.

16h. (B) After the initial replacement with isotonic saline, hypotonic saline (0.45%), which is similar to fluid lost during osmotic diuresis, is administered to replace water lost from both intracellular and extracellular spaces.

16i. (E) Initial fluid replacement in DKA patients is usually devoid of additives. Subsequent fluid replacement solutions usually contain potassium and phosphorus as these tend to decline as therapy is initiated. Protocols typically indicate replacing potassium as 2/3 potassium chloride and 1/3 potassium phosphate or as equal proportions of each.

16j. (C) Bicarbonate is no longer recommended in the routine management of DKA. Several disadvantages of bicarbonate include worsened hypokalemia, production of paradoxical central nervous system acidosis, worsened intracellular acidosis, and prolongation of ketoanion metabolism. Bicarbonate may be considered if the patient's arterial pH is < 7.0.

16k. (C) Regular insulin is available as a solution and is the only insulin indicated to be administered via intravenous infusion.

16l. (B) The recommended initial insulin infusion dose in the treatment of DKA is 0.1 u/kg/hr. Therefore, for Nell, 0.1 u/kg/hr × 55 kg = 5.5 u/hr.

16m. (C) Nell is prescribed 10 u/hr. Therefore, 10 u/hr × 24 hours = 240 u/day. Insulin is available as 100 u/mL, therefore, 100 u/mL = 240 u/x; x = 2.4 mL.

16n. (A) During the treatment of DKA, the major potassium-lowering effect is insulin mediated reentry of potassium to the intracellular compartment. Extracellular fluid volume expansion and resolution of acidemia play a role as well. During early treatment, there is a continued negative potassium balance because of ongoing osmotic diuresis and ketonuria.

16o. (D) A continuous supply of insulin is needed to prevent ketosis and permit continued anabolism. Therefore, in lieu of decreasing the insulin infusion, serum glucose concentrations should be maintained at desired concentrations by the addition of dextrose to maintenance fluids.

CASE 17

17a. (E) Hypoplastic left heart syndrome (HLHS) occurs in ~ 1% of all congenital heart defects and is the most common cause of death from cardiac defects during the first month of life. It includes a group of closely related anomalies including hypoplasia of the left ventricle, atresia or stenosis of the aortic arch and/or mitral valves, and hypoplasia of the ascending aorta and aortic arch. Coarctation of the aorta is present in ~ 75% of cases. An atrial and/or ventricular septal defect may also be present.

17b. (D) The two surgical options for HLHS are a Norwood operation followed by a Fontan or a cardiac transplantation.

17c. (A) The administration of loop diuretics may result in a hypochloremic metabolic alkalosis. A low serum chloride and an elevated serum bicarbonate are indicative of such a metabolic disturbance.

17d. (A) Daniel's serum potassium is low which may be a result of his diuretic therapy. Potassium supplementation should be prescribed for Daniel with subsequent close monitoring of his serum potassium concentration.

17e. (B) Given Daniel's low ionized calcium concentration (normal ~ 1.1–1.3 mMol/L), it would be prudent to administer a bolus dose of intravenous calcium gluconate 100 mg/kg. Calcium carbonate is only available in oral dosage forms. The correct dose of intravenous calcium chloride is 10 mg/kg.

17f. (B) Normal serum-ionized calcium concentration ranges from ~ 1.1–1.3 mMol/L. Therefore, a concentration of 1.12 mMol/L would be acceptable.

17g. (C) Intravenous pressor agents are often prepared using the "rule of 6." Using this rule, an arbitrary "N" factor is multiplied by the patient's weight and then multiplied by 6. This product is the amount of drug in milligrams that should be added per 100 mL of final solution. Of this preparation, for each 1 mL/hr infused, the patient receives N mcg/kg/min of drug. In this example (N = 5, weight = 4.5 kg, rate = 2 mL/hr), 5 × 4.5 × 6 = 135. Therefore, 135 mg of dopamine would be included in each 100 mL of final product. With a rate of 2 mL/hr, the patient would be receiving N × 2 mcg/kg/min or 5 × 2 = 10 mcg/kg/min of dopamine.

17h. (B) Nitrogard, Nitro-Dur, and Nitrostat are nitroglycerin products. Nitropress is nitroprusside.

17i. (B) Nitroprusside is a direct-acting vasodilator used in the treatment of hypertensive crisis and also as an afterload reducer.

17j. (B) Nitroprusside consists of five cyanide molecules per nitroprusside molecule that are released in-vivo, and therefore have the potential to result in cyanide toxicity.

17k. (A) One of the cyanide molecules reacts with met-hemoglobin to produce cyanomethemoglobin. The remaining four molecules of cyanide are converted to thiocyanate by thiosulfate in the presence of the mitochondrial enzyme rhodanese. The rate-limiting factor is thiosulfate of which may be inadequate with excessive doses of nitroprusside. Therefore, administering sodium thiosulfate in a concentration of 10:1 with nitroprusside protects against nitroprusside-induced cyanide toxicity.

17l. (A) Nitroprusside solutions should be protected from light during administration to prevent product degradation. A discolored solution indicates drug breakdown and should be discarded. Nitroprusside is only administered parenterally with a usual dosing range being between 1–5 mcg/kg/min.

17m. (A) The respective trade and generic names are: Primacor (milrinone), Inocor (amrinone), Dobutrex (dobutamine), and Adrenalin (epinephrine).

17n. (A) Milrinone and amrinone are both inotropes/vasodilators that exert their effects through inhibition of phosphodiesterases.

17o. (C)

17p. (C) Renal clearance of unchanged parent drug accounts for ~ 85% of total body clearance of milrinone. Unlike pressor agents such as dopamine and norepinephrine that have half-lives of only a few minutes, the half-life of milrinone is ~ 2 hours. Because of its β-adrenergic effects, milrinone is beneficial to patients suffering from congestive heart failure.

17q. (B) Due to its longer half-life, milrinone therapy is often initiated with a loading dose of 50–75 mcg/kg followed by an infusion up to 1 mcg/kg/min.

17r. (D) Pediatric dosing of ketorolac includes 0.5–1 mg/kg iv q 6 hours. Since dosing should not exceed 5 days, a stop date should be included in the initial order.

CASE 18

18a. (E) Tetralogy of Fallot (TOF) classically includes the following four anomalies: A large ventricular septal defect (VSD), right ventricular (RV) outflow tract obstruction, right ventricular hypertrophy (RVH), and an overriding of the aorta.

18b. (E) Cyanotic spells, known as hypoxic or tet spells, manifest as hyperpnea, irritability, prolonged crying, increasing cyanosis, and decreasing intensity of the heart murmur. The peak incidence of hypoxic spells is between 2–4 months of age.

18c. (B) Morphine sulfate is used in the treatment of cyanotic spells to suppress the respiratory center and abolish hyperpnea.

18d. (E) Morphine sulfate is available for oral, intravenous, intramuscular, and subcutaneous administration. The parenteral route is preferred for treating hypoxic spells.

18e. (A) Sodium bicarbonate 8.4% = 8.4 gms/100 mL or 8400 mg/100 mL; 1 mEq sodium bicarbonate = 84 mg; prescribed dose = 1 mEq/kg = 1 mEq × 5 kg = 5 mEq; 1 mEq/84 mg = 5 mEq/x; x = 420 mg; so 8400 mg/100 mL = 420 mg/x; x = 5 mL.

18f. (D) Sodium bicarbonate is a hypertonic solution that may result in tissue necrosis subsequent to extravasation. Due to its sodium content, caution is warranted when administering to congestive heart failure patients or those with other sodium retaining problems. Sodium bicarbonate dissociates to provide bicarbonate to neutralize hydrogen ion concentrations.

18g. (B) The respective trade and generic names are: Visken (pindolol), Inderal (propranolol), Tenormin (atenolol), and Lopressor (metoprolol).

18h. (D) Propranolol is a non-selective beta adrenergic antagonist, and therefore reacts with both β-1 and β-2 receptors.

18i. (A). The maximum recommended dose of intravenous propranolol for an infant and child is 1 and 3 mg, respectively.

18j. (C) Dose = 0.05 mg × 5 kg = 0.25 mg; 0.01% solution = 0.01 g/100 mL or 1 mg/10 mL; 1 mg/10 mL = 0.25 mg/x; x = 2.5 mL.

18k. (E) A vasoconstrictor, such as phenylephrine (Neo-Synephrine), may also be effective for the treatment of cyanotic spells. Ketamine may also be helpful as it increases systemic vascular resistance and provides sedation.

18l. (B) Oral propranolol may be used to prevent the recurrence of cyanotic spells and to delay corrective surgical procedures in high-risk patients.

CASE 19

19a. (E) Interrupted aortic arch is usually associated with a patent ductus arteriosus (PDA) and ventricular septal defect (VSD). With a Type B interruption, Di George syndrome is reported in ~ 50% of patients.

19b. (C) Ventricular septal defect is the most common form of congenital heart defect (CHD) and accounts for ~ 20% of all CHDs. Infants with a small VSD are well-developed and acyanotic. Delayed growth and development, decreased exercise tolerance, repeated pulmonary infections, and congestive heart failure are common during infancy in the presence of a moderate to large VSD. Treatment of VSD and associated CHF is with digoxin and diuretics for 2–4 months in an attempt to improve growth failure. Frequent feedings with high calorie formulas may be helpful. Iron therapy may be used to correct anemia. Maintaining good dental hygiene is important. If growth failure is not improved by medical therapy, the VSD should be surgically repaired within the first 6 months of life.

19c. (E) Digoxin inhibits sarcolemmal sodium-potassium-ATPase to enhance contractility via increasing intracellular calcium concentrations leading to an increase in the force of myocardial contractions (positive inotrope). Digoxin is a negative chronotrope and decreases conduction through the sinoatrial and atrioventricular nodes.

19d. (A) Hypokalemia increases the myocardium's sensitivity to digoxin and may lead to toxic manifestations of digoxin.

19e. (B) The digitalizing or loading of digoxin is usually performed by administering one-half of the loading dose followed by the remaining half in two equal doses at 6 to 12 hour intervals. ECG's are often monitored during loading to assess for toxicity.

19f. (B) The accepted therapeutic serum concentration of digoxin is between 0.8–2 ng/mL. Concentrations approaching the upper therapeutic range are often needed to resolve arrhythmias whereas lower concentrations may be sufficient in the treatment of CHF.

19g. (D) The distribution or alpha phase of digoxin is delayed and therefore concentrations should be obtained at least 6 hours after dosing.

19h. (B) The bioavailability of digoxin liquid filled capsules, elixir, and tablets is 90–100%, 70–85%, and 60–80%, respectively.

19i. (E) The presence of endogenous digoxin like immunoreactive substances (EDLIS) give rise to falsely elevated digoxin concentrations and have been identified during pregnancy, in children younger than 6 years old, and in patients with renal or hepatic dysfunction.

19j. (D) Some labs are equipped with columns that remove EDLIS and are able to report a "true" digoxin concentration. In the absence of such equipment, patients with possible EDLIS should be monitored clinically for signs of toxicity (i.e., ECG).

19k. (C) Although 0.13 mL of the stock solution is the correct amount for the prescribed dose (100 mcg/mL = 13 mcg/x; x = 0.13 mL), the accuracy of measuring such a small dose of a critical drug should be questioned. Therefore, it would be prudent to prepare a dilution so that a larger volume may be measured. Diluting 1 mL (100 mcg) to a total of 5 mL would provide 100 mcg/5mLs. Therefore, 100 mcg/5 mL = 13 mcg/x; x = 0.65 mL.

19l. (A) Digoxin immune fab (Digibind) binds to unbound digoxin or digitoxin that is then removed by renal excretion.

19m. (B) The recommended initial dose of alprostadil is 0.05–0.1 mcg/kg/min. Maintenance doses are usually between 0.01 to 0.4 mcg/kg/min.

19n. (B) Spironolactone is a potassium-sparing diuretic and therefore, may increase serum potassium concentrations.

19o. (C) The bioavailability of furosemide is ~ 50%. Therefore, when converting from intravenous to oral therapy, doubling of the dose is often required to obtain the same diuretic effect.

19p. (C) With normal renal function, as in James' case,

vancomycin should be initially dosed at 15–20 mg/kg every 8 hours.

19q. (D) Coagulase negative *Staphylococcus* is a gram-positive bacteria that is sensitive to vancomycin. Therefore, in the absence of gram-negative sepsis, the ceftazidime may be discontinued.

CASE 20

20a. (A) Although not well established, pediatric doses of sucralfate (Carafate) typically range from 40–80 mg/kg/day. Therefore, Chris might receive 100 mg po q 6 h (400 mg/day/7.5 kg = 53 mg/kg/day).

20b. (D) Sucralfate is a aluminum salt of sulfated sucrose that forms a paste-like substance in the gastric acidic environment and subsequently adheres to damaged mucosa.

20c. (C) Unasyn is a combination product containing a penicillin (ampicillin) and β-lactamase inhibitor (sulbactam).

20d. (C) Each 1.5 grams of Unasyn contains 1 gram of ampicillin (major antibacterial component) and 500 mg of sulbactam. Therefore, Unasyn is ~ 67% ampicillin. Therefore, Chris' dose of 350mg contains ~ 234 mg of ampicillin (350 mg × 0.67 = 234 mg).

20e. (B) Prograf is the trade name for tacrolimus of which FK-506 is a synonym. Neoral and Sandimmune are cyclosporine products. CellCept is the trade name for mycophenolate mofetil.

20f. (C) Inhibition of calcineurin activity by the FK-506-FK-binding protein complex inhibits the transcription of genes for interleukin-2, interleukin-3, interleukin-4, granulocyte-macrophage colony-stimulating factor, tumor necrosis factor-alpha, and gamma-interferon-cytokines involved in the early phase of T-cell activation.

20g. (C) The mean bioavailability of FK-506 is ~ 30% (range 5–67%) and is unaffected by the presence of bile acids. FK-506 is found in high concentrations in the lungs, spleen, heart, kidney, pancreas, brain, muscle, and liver. It is hepatically metabolized by the cytochrome P-450 isoenzyme system to at least nine metabolites with less than 1% of the dose excreted in the urine as unchanged drug.

20h. (A) Therapeutic trough concentrations of FK-506 have been reported as 10–20 ng/mL in whole blood and 0.5–2 ng/mL in plasma.

20i. (B) The initial mean dose of intravenous FK-506 for pediatric patients is typically 0.1 mg/kg/day as an infusion.

20j. (C) A reasonable initial oral dose of FK-506 for a pediatric patient would be 0.3 mg/kg/day in two divided doses (0.15 mg/kg/dose).

20k. (D) The mean half-life of FK-506 is approximately 10 hours. With 4–5 half-lives needed to reach a new steady-state concentration, ~ 50 hours (5 half-lives × 10 hours = 50 hours) should elapse before reassessing Chris' FK-506 concentration after his dosage change.

20l. (E) Since FK-506 is metabolized by the cytochrome P-450 isoenzyme system, drugs that inhibit this metabolic pathway could potentially cause increased FK-506 concentrations. Diltiazem, ketoconazole, and fluconazole are all inhibitors of the cytochrome P-450 isoenzyme system and may increase FK-506 concentrations.

20m. (E) Complications of FK-506 therapy include nephrotoxicity, hyperkalemia, infections, neurotoxicity, glucose intolerance, hypertension, hypercholesterolemia, hirsutism, and gingival hyperplasia.

20n. (A) Chris' daily dose = 0.3 mg/kg/day × 7.5 kg = 2.25 mg/day or 1.13 mg per 12 hours. Therefore, 5 mg/mL = 1.13 mg/x; x = 0.23 mL.

20o. (E) In the event rejection is suspected, other immunosuppressants such as OKT3, azathioprine, or higher doses of corticosteroids may be prescribed.

20p. (B) Cyclosporine is an immunosuppressant agent with a mechanism of action similar to FK-506. Generally, in liver transplant patients, FK-506 appears to be a more favorable agent regarding efficacy and adverse effects.

Pediatric In-Patient

*Ignorance is only dangerous
when it is not realized*

This section consists of 18 medication orders followed by corresponding patient profiles representing pharmacotherapy associated with patients admitted to a hospital's general pediatric ward. Each patient profile is followed by multiple-choice questions pertaining to the medication order and profile information. Choose the one best-lettered response to each item. The correct answers are provided at the end of this section. The reader is encouraged to attempt all questions for each case or for the entire section before referring to the answer key. Moreover, where appropriate, the answer key provides an explanation of the correct response and should serve as an additional learning tool for the reader.

CASE 1

PHYSICIAN ORDER

Patient Weight: 11 kg

IVIG 11 grams iv × 1 dose
Aspirin 110 mg po q 6 hours

Date/Time: 11/12/0900
Physician: John Small

Patient Name: Tina Reeves
Patient ID #: 213230

MEDICAL PROFILE

Patient: Tina Reeves

Patient Weight: 11 kg   **Age:** 13 m/o

Present Illness: Possible Kawasaki Syndrome

Allergies: None

Medical History: Unremarkable

Labs: Na 136, K 3.7, Cl 110, C02 21, Cr 0.4, BUN 6, Glu 97, Mg 2.1, WBC 9700, H/H 7.8/25.6, Plat 682,000, Segs 38%, Bands 12%, Lymphs 2%, Monos 1%, CRP 12.4

Vitals Name: B/P 110/70, P 120, R 20, T 40 C

Cultures: Pending

ECHO: Pending

Medication Profile:

Date	Medication
11/12/0830	Cefotaxime 550 mg iv q 8 h

1a. Which of the following is true regarding Kawasaki Syndrome (KS)?

   A. Rarely occurs in patients younger than 8 years of age
   B. Occurs more commonly in children of Japanese and Korean decent
   C. Girls are affected more often than boys
   D. A and B only
   E. A, B, and C

1b. Which of the following is a proposed etiology of KS?

   A. Retrovirus
   B. Toxin of Propionibacterium acnes
   C. Toxic shock syndrome toxin producing *Staphylococcus*
   D. A and B only
   E. A, B, and C

1c. The most concerning manifestation of KS is the associated _____.

A. liver failure
B. vasculitis of the coronary blood vessels
C. aseptic meningitis
D. fever

1d. The diagnostic criteria for KS include _____.

A. fever of at least 3 days duration
B. truncal rash
C. cervical lymphadenopathy
D. B and C only
E. A, B, and C

1e. Which of Tina's laboratory values is consistent with KS?

A. WBC
B. Platelets
C. CRP
D. A and C only
E. A, B, and C

1f. A goal in the management of KS is to _____.

A. alter the inflammatory process
B. prevent coronary artery involvement
C. inhibit platelet aggregation
D. A and B only
E. A, B, and C

1g. Which of the following is a trade name for intravenous immune globulin (IVIG)?

A. Venoglobulin-S
B. Gamimune
C. Sandoglobulin
D. A and B only
E. A, B, and C

1h. A possible adverse effect of IVIG includes

_____.

A. hypotension
B. flushing
C. chest tightness
D. A and B only
E. A, B, and C

1i. A more appropriate dose of IVIG for Tina would be

_____.

A. 11 gms iv qd × 2 days
B. 22 gms iv qd × 1 day
C. 22 gms iv qd × 2 days
D. 4.4 gms iv qd × 1 day

1j. Which of the following would be the most appropriate infusion time over which to administer Tina's IVIG?

A. 5 minutes
B. 1 hour
C. 2 hours
D. 12 hours

1k. Which of the following is a pharmacological effect associated with aspirin therapy?

A. Antipyretic
B. Anti-inflammatory
C. Analgesic
D. A and C only
E. A, B, and C

1l. Which of the following is an adverse effect associated with aspirin therapy?

A. Gastrointestinal bleeding
B. Peptic ulcer
C. Bronchospasms
D. A and B only
E. A, B, and C

1m. Which of the following is true regarding the disposition of aspirin during the acute phase of KS?

A. There appears to be a decrease in unbound salicylate concentrations
B. Excessive doses are often required to achieve therapeutic concentrations
C. There appears to be decreased absorption and increased clearance
D. B and C only
E. A, B, and C

1n. A reasonable targeted aspirin serum concentration during the acute phase of KS would be _____.

A. 1–5 mg/dL
B. 5–10 mg/dL
C. 5–10 mg/L
D. 20–25 mg/dL

1o. A more appropriate aspirin regimen for Tina would be _____.

A. 81 mg po q 8 hours
B. 162 mg po q 8 hours
C. 162 mg po q 6 hours
D. 243 mg po q 6 hours

1p. In the absence of fever, at approximately the 14th day after the onset of KS, it would be prudent to decrease Tina's aspirin dose to _____.

   A. 40 mg po qd
   B. 81 mg po qd
   C. 163 mg po qd
   D. 325 mg po qd

1q. In the event that Tina acquires a viral infection while on aspirin therapy, an appropriate action would be to _____.

   A. decrease her daily dose by one-half
   B. decrease her daily dose by one-half and prescribe dipyridamole
   C. discontinue her aspirin therapy and prescribe dipyridamole
   D. maintain her same aspirin dose and prescribe dipyridamole

1r. Long-term pharmacologic therapy for Tina might include the use of _____.

   A. aspirin
   B. dipyridamole
   C. warfarin
   D. A and B only
   E. A, B, and C

CASE 2

PHYSICIAN ORDER

Patient Weight: 25 kg

Azithromycin 125 mg iv qd

Date/Time: 2/29/0900   **Patient Name:** John Sawyer
Physician: Jeff Cook   **Patient ID #:** 983230

MEDICAL PROFILE

Patient: John Sawyer   **Patient Weight:** 25 kg   **Age:** 7 y/o

Present Illness: Bilateral pneumonia   **Allergies:** None

Medical History: Unremarkable

Labs: Na 137, K 5.1, Cl 103, C02 23, Cr 0.4, BUN 5, Glu 92, Ca 9, WBC 18000, H/H 11/33.7, Plat 751,000, Segs 46%, Bands 4%, Lymphs 34%, Monos 16%, CRP 6.5, vancomycin peak and trough conc's: 2/29/0600 = 18, 2/29/1200 = 4.5

Cultures: Pending (blood and sputum)

Medication Profile:

Date	Medication
2/28/0900	Acetaminophen 250 mg po q 4–6 h prn
2/28/0900	Vancomycin 350 mg iv q 8 h
2/28/0900	Rocephin 1250 mg iv bid

2a. The most common bacterial pathogen associated with community-acquired pneumonia in children is

_____.

   A. *Haemophilus influenzae*
   B. *Streptococcus pneumoniae*
   C. *Mycoplasma pneumoniae*
   D. *Moraxella catarrhalis*

2b. Antibiotic resistance to which of the following bacteria would most likely be overcome by administering higher doses of antibiotics?

   A. *Haemophilus influenzae*
   B. *Streptococcus pneumoniae*
   C. Methicillin-resistant *Staphylococcus aureus*
   D. A and B only
   E. A, B, and C

2c. A mechanism by which *Streptococcus pneumoniae* develops resistance to the macrolides includes

_____.

   A. alteration of the 30S ribosome
   B. the presence of efflux pumps
   C. altered penicillin binding sites
   D. A and B only
   E. A, B, and C

2d. The generic name for Rocephin is _____.

   A. cefotaxime
   B. ceftazidime
   C. cefoxitin
   D. ceftriaxone

2e. Rocephin is classified as a _____ generation cephalosporin.

  A. first-
  B. second-
  C. third-
  D. fourth-

2f. The mechanism of action of Rocephin involves inhibition of _____.

  A. bacterial protein synthesis
  B. viral protein synthesis
  C. bacterial cell-wall synthesis
  D. viral cell-wall synthesis

2g. Which of the following pathogens is typically susceptible to Rocephin?

  A. *Streptococcus pneumoniae*
  B. *Haemophilus influenzae*
  C. *Mycoplasma pneumoniae*
  D. A and B only
  E. A, B, and C

2h. The appropriate dose of Rocephin for John is _____.

  A. 625 mg iv qd
  B. 625 mg iv bid
  C. 1250 mg iv qd
  D. 1250 mg iv bid

2i. The maximum recommended daily dose of Rocephin for a 50-kg child would be _____ grams.

  A. two
  B. three
  C. four
  D. five

2j. Vancomycin was most likely added to John's regimen for additional coverage against _____.

  A. anaerobic bacteria
  B. *Haemophilus influenzae*
  C. *Streptococcus pneumoniae*
  D. *Mycoplasma pneumoniae*

2k. John's vancomycin half-life is _____ hours.

  A. 2
  B. 3
  C. 4
  D. 6

2l. A reasonable targeted vancomycin trough concentration for John would be _____.

  A. 1–5 mg/L
  B. 1–5 mcg/L
  C. 5–10 mg/L
  D. 5–10 mcg/L

2m. A more appropriate initial dose of vancomycin for John would be _____.

  A. 250 mg iv q 8 h
  B. 500 mg iv q 8 h
  C. 500 mg iv q 6 h
  D. 1 gm iv q 12 h

2n. Red Man Syndrome is associated with which of the following medications?

  A. Ceftriaxone
  B. Vancomycin
  C. Azithromycin
  D. Cefotaxime

2o. The trade name for azithromycin is _____.

  A. Zithromax
  B. Biaxin
  C. E-mycin
  D. Zyban

2p. Azithromycin is typically referred to as a(n) _____.

  A. penicillin
  B. cephalosporin
  C. macrolide
  D. atypical

2q. The mechanism of action of azithromycin involves inhibition of bacterial _____.

  A. cell-wall synthesis
  B. protein synthesis by binding to the 30 S ribosome
  C. protein synthesis by binding to the 50 S ribosome
  D. sterol production

2r. Which of the following would have been a reasonable alternative for azithromycin for John?

  A. Clindamycin
  B. Clarithromycin
  C. Gentamicin
  D. Ganciclovir

2s. Azithromycin was most likely prescribed to John for the treatment of possible _____.

    A. *Staphylococcus aureus*
    B. *Haemophilus influenzae*
    C. *Streptococcus pyogenes*
    D. *Mycoplasma pneumoniae*

2t. A more appropriate dose of azithromycin for John would be _____.

    A. 125 mg iv bid
    B. 250 mg iv qd
    C. 250 mg iv bid
    D. 500 mg iv qd

CASE 3

PHYSICIAN ORDER

Patient Weight: <u>17 kg</u>

Discontinue azithromycin
Add cefotaxime 850 mg iv q 8 hours

Date/Time: <u>05/13/1600</u>
Physician: <u>Sam Birch</u>

Patient Name: <u>Bobby Rhine</u>
Patient ID #: <u>783230</u>

MEDICAL PROFILE

Patient: Bobby Rhine

Patient Weight: 17 kg **Age:** 4 y/o

Present Illness: Aspiration pneumonia

Allergies: Ampicillin (diarrhea)

Medical History: Epilepsy

Labs: Na 139, K 4.1, Cl 107, C02 22, Cr 0.5, BUN 8, Glu 89, Mg 1.9, WBC 10200, H/H 12.4/35.6, Plat 229,000, Segs 71%, Bands 23%, Lymphs 3%, Monos 1%, CRP 5.9

Cultures: Endotracheal aspirate (pending); Mycoplasma IgG negative; IgM negative

Medication Profile:

Date	Medication
5/12/0800	Azithromycin 170 mg iv qd
5/12/0800	Timentin 1250 mg iv q 12 h
5/12/0800	Albuterol 2.5 mg neb q 4 h
5/12/0800	Acetaminophen 175 mg po q 4 h prn
5/12/0800	Carbamazepine 150 mg po tid

3a. Which of the following is associated with aspiration pneumonia?

A. Decreased level of consciousness
B. Epilepsy
C. Dysphagia
D. A and B only
E. A, B, and C

3b. The normal oral flora consists of _____.

A. *Bacteroides*
B. *Streptococci*
C. *Fusobacterium*
D. A and B only
E. A, B, and C

3c. The oropharynx of hospitalized patients is often colonized with _____.

A. *Klebsiella*
B. *Pseudomonas*
C. *Staphylococcus*
D. A and B only
E. A, B, and C

3d. A reliable technique to detect the presence of bacteria for suspected aspiration pneumonia involves the use of _____.

A. blood cultures
B. brush cultures
C. expectorated sputum
D. A and B only
E. A, B, and C

3e. Which of the following was the most likely reason for the discontinuation of azithromycin in Bobby?

A. The negative IgG result
B. His elevated percentage of bands
C. His elevated white blood cell count
D. The negative IgM result

3f. The brand name of cefotaxime is _____.

A. Rocephin
B. Fortaz
C. Suprax
D. Claforan

3g. Cefotaxime is classified as a _____ generation cephalosporin.

A. first-
B. second-
C. third-
D. fourth-

3h. Which of the following statements is most accurate regarding the prescribing of cefotaxime to Bobby?

A. Provides increased anaerobic coverage
B. Allows enhanced coverage against *Mycoplasma*
C. Acts synergistically with Timentin
D. Most likely provides no additional benefit

3i. Timentin was prescribed to Bobby because of its activity against _____.

A. gram-positive bacteria
B. gram-negative bacteria
C. anaerobes
D. A and B only
E. A, B, and C

3j. A more appropriate dosage of Timentin for Bobby would be _____.

A. 850 mg iv q 8 h
B. 850 mg iv q 6 h
C. 1250 mg iv q 12 h
D. 1250 mg iv q 6 h

3k. The most concerning toxic effect from an overdose of Timentin is _____.

A. pseudomembranous colitis
B. seizures
C. renal failure
D. hyperkalemia

3l. Timentin contains a high content of which of the following?

A. Potassium
B. Sodium
C. Magnesium
D. Phosphorus

3m. The maximum recommended single dose of Timentin is _____.

A. 3 grams
B. 3.1 grams
C. 3.2 grams
D. 3.3 grams

3n. Which of the following would be an appropriate alternative to Timentin to prescribe to Bobby?

A. Zosyn
B. Nebcin
C. Cleocin
D. Ceclor

3o. Which of the following would be an appropriate suggestion to make to Dr. Birch regarding Bobby's documented allergy?

A. Administer diphenhydramine prior to each Timentin dose
B. Do not prescribe cefotaxime
C. Desensitize Bobby during his first dose of cefotaxime
D. Remove the documented allergy from Bobby's medical record

CASE 4

PHYSICIAN ORDER

Patient Weight: <u>60 kg</u>

ADEK 2 tabs po qd
Pancrease MT 16 4 caps with meals and 2 caps with snacks

Date/Time: <u>9/11/0900</u>
Physician: <u>Matthew Morrison</u>

Patient Name: <u>Heath Crisp</u>
Patient ID #: <u>897677</u>

MEDICAL PROFILE

Patient: Heath Crisp

Patient Weight: 60 kg   **Age:** 16 y/o

Present Illness: Fever, possible sepsis

Allergies: None

Medical History: Cystic fibrosis

Labs: Na 135, K 3.8, Cl 105, C02 22.9, Cr 0.6, BUN 9, Glu 78, WBC 14300, H/H 14.7/44.3, Plat 340,000, Segs 56%, Bands 9%, Lymphs 21%, Monos 14%, CRP 8.6, Alk Phos 188, ALT 45, AST 32, Total Bili 0.9, Direct Bili 0.1, Total Protein 7.6, Alb 3.1, PTT 31.6, PT 14.8, Tobramycin: 9/11/0500 = 5; 9/11/1130 = 0.5

Cultures: Tracheal aspirate – *Staphylococcus aureus* (sensitivities pending)

Medication Profile:

Date	Medication
9/10/1100	Tobramycin 120 mg iv q 8 h
9/10/1100	Vancomycin 1 gram iv q 12 h
9/10/1100	Pulmozyme 1.5 ml qd
9/10/1100	Albuterol 2.5 mg neb q 4 h
9/10/1100	Tobi 40 mg

4a. Which of the following is true regarding cystic fibrosis?

   A. Is associated with a defect in a gene on chromosome 9
   B. The associated gene mutation affects the c-AMP regulated chloride channel termed the CFTR
   C. The most common gene mutation is the delta F-508 and accounts for approximately 70% of mutant cystic fibrosis alleles
   D. B and C only
   E. A, B, and C

4b. Cystic fibrosis is associated with
_____.

   A. elevated sweat chloride concentrations
   B. pulmonary infections
   C. pancreatic insufficiency
   D. A and B only
   E. A, B, and C

4c. During infancy, which of the following conditions prompt consideration for the diagnosis of cystic fibrosis?

A. Prolonged jaundice
B. Failure to thrive
C. Meconium ileus
D. A and B only
E. A, B, and C

4d. Which of the following is indicative of cystic fibrosis?

A. Sweat chloride concentration greater than 60 mEq/L
B. Recurrent or persistent pulmonary infections
C. Fatty stools
D. B and C only
E. A, B, and C

4e. Which of the following bacteria is more predominant as cystic fibrosis progresses?

A. *Staphylococcus*
B. *Haemophilus*
C. *Pseudomonas*
D. A and B only
E. A, B, and C

4f. The Nebcin was most likely prescribed for Heath for the treatment of possible _____.

A. *Staphylococcus*
B. *Streptococcus*
C. *Pseudomonas*
D. *Candida*

4g. A reasonable initial dose of tobramycin for Heath would be _____.

A. 1 mg/kg iv q 8 h
B. 1.5 mg/kg iv q 8 h
C. 2 mg/kg iv q 8 h
D. 3 mg/kg iv q 8 h

4h. The calculated tobramycin half-life for Heath is approximately _____ hour(s).

A. 1
B. 2
C. 3
D. 4

4i. What dose of tobramycin should be prescribed to Heath to attain a peak concentration of ~ 7.5 mcg/mL?

A. 130 mg iv q 8 h
B. 140 mg iv q 8 h
C. 160 mg iv q 8 h
D. 180 mg iv q 8 h

4j. Pending bacterial sensitivities, which of the following would be the most appropriate alternative to vancomycin therapy?

A. Cefotaxime
B. Oxacillin
C. Aztreonam
D. Azithromycin

4k. An alternative name for Pulmozyme is _____.

A. DNase
B. dornase alfa
C. recombinant human deoxyribonuclease
D. A and B only
E. A, B, and C

4l. The mechanism of action of Pulmozyme involves _____.

A. bronchodilation
B. hydrolyzing DNA in respiratory secretions
C. mast-cell stabilization
D. inhibition of acetylcholine

4m. The correct dose of nebulized Pulmozyme for Heath is _____.

A. 1.5 mg qd
B. 2 mg qd
C. 2.5 mg qd
D. 3 mg qd

4n. Which of the following is true of the ADEK prescribed for Heath?

A. Contains only vitamins A, D, E, and K
B. Correct dose for Heath is 2 tablets orally daily
C. Tablets should be swallowed whole (i.e., not crushed or chewed)
D. A and C only
E. A, B, and C

4o. Pancrease is dosed based on the amount of _____ present in the formulation.

A. amylase
B. protease
C. lipase
D. DNase

4p. Each Pancrease capsule prescribed for Heath contains what quantity of the component referred to in question 4o?

A. 16 units
B. 160 units
C. 1600 units
D. 16,000 units

4q. Excessive dosing of Pancrease may result in _____.

A. constipation
B. mucosal irritation
C. colonic strictures
D. A and B only
E. A, B, and C

CASE 5

PHYSICIAN ORDER

Patient Weight: <u>15 kg</u>

Discontinue imipenem/cilastatin
Begin meropenem 150 mg q 6 h

Date/Time: <u>3/25/1400</u>
Physician: <u>Mike Toms</u>

Patient Name: <u>Daryl Stevens</u>
Patient ID #: <u>963230</u>

MEDICAL PROFILE

Patient: Daryl Stevens

Present Illness: Right lower pneumonia

Patient Weight: 15 kg   **Age:** 3 y/o

Allergies: Ceclor, has received other cephalosporins without incidence

Medical History: Tonsillectomy and adenoidectomy, seizures

Labs: Na 138, K 4.1, Cl 108, C02 22, Cr 0.5, BUN 7, Glu 105, Mg 2.2, WBC 14500, H/H 12.7/37.5, Plat 250,000, Segs 70%, Bands 24%, Lymphs 3%, Monos 2%, CRP 16

Cultures: Pending

Medication Profile:

Date	Medication
3/24/1500	Acetaminophen 225 mg po q 6 h prn
3/24/1500	Acetaminophen with codeine 3 mLs q 4–6 h prn
3/24/1500	Imipenem/cilastatin 225 mg iv q 6 h
3/24/1500	Vancomycin 300 mg iv q 8 h
3/24/1500	Phenytoin 25 mg po q 8 h

5a. How many milliliters of Tylenol 160 mg/5 mL are needed to provide Daryl with his prescribed dose?

A. 3.5
B. 5
C. 6.5
D. 7

5b. How many milligrams of codeine will Daryl receive with each of his prescribed doses of acetaminophen with codeine?

A. 5.1 mg
B. 7.2 mg
C. 10.1 mg
D. 14.7 mg

5c. How many milligrams of acetaminophen will Daryl receive with each of his prescribed doses of acetaminophen with codeine?

A. 51 mg
B. 72 mg
C. 101 mg
D. 147 mg

5d. Imipenem/cilastatin belongs to a class of medications known as the _____.

A. macrolides
B. cephalosporins
C. carbapenems
D. penicillins

5e. The trade name for imipenem/cilastatin is _____.

    A. Primaxin
    B. Prinivil
    C. Pentam
    D. Principen

5f. Which of the following bacteria is usually susceptible to imipenem/cilastatin?

    A. Gram-positives
    B. Gram-negatives
    C. Anaerobes
    D. A and B only
    E. A, B, and C

5g. The role of cilastatin as a component of imipenem/cilastatin is to prevent the _____.

    A. hepatic metabolism of imipenem
    B. renal metabolism of imipenem
    C. degradation of imipenem by penicillinase
    D. degradation of imipenem by hydrochloric acid

5h. The maximum recommended daily dose of imipenem/cilastatin is ____ grams.

    A. 2
    B. 4
    C. 6
    D. 8

5i. Imipenem/cilastatin may not be an appropriate medication for Daryl because of his _____.

    A. elevated serum creatinine
    B. diagnosis of pneumonia
    C. concurrent vancomycin therapy
    D. history of seizures

5j. The trade name of meropenem is _____.

    A. Mavik
    B. Merrem
    C. Maxipime
    D. Miltown

5k. Which of the following is true of meropenem?

    A. Dosage adjustments are needed in the presence of renal dysfunction
    B. Is not indicated for the treatment of meningitis
    C. Maximum recommended daily dose is 3 grams
    D. A and B only
    E. A, B, and C

5l. Which of the following bacteria is usually susceptible to meropenem?

    A. Gram-positive
    B. Gram-negative
    C. MRSA
    D. A and B only
    E. A, B, and C

5m. Which of the following is true regarding Daryl's meropenem order?

    A. The dose should be altered
    B. The dosing interval should be altered
    C. Both the dose and dosing interval should be altered
    D. Neither the dose or dosing interval should be altered

5n. Daryl's meropenem should be administered via what route?

    A. PO
    B. IM
    C. IV
    D. IM or IV

5o. Which of the following might explain Daryl's reaction to Ceclor?

    A. First-generation allergic syndrome
    B. Serum sickness
    C. Reaction to additive or flavoring agent
    D. Inactivation by bacteria

CASE 6

PHYSICIAN ORDER

Patient Weight: 18 kg

Discontinue ceftazidime and oxacillin
Vancomycin 360 mg iv q 8 h. Obtain peak and trough with 3rd dose

Date/Time: 5/22/1500
Physician: Todd Manus

Patient Name: Susan Tisdale
Patient ID #: 852698

MEDICAL PROFILE

Patient: Susan Tisdale

Patient Weight: 18 kg   **Age:** 7 y/o

Present Illness: Sepsis

Allergies: None

Medical History: End stage renal disease

Labs: Na 142, K 5.3, Cl 112, C02 19, Cr 12.7, BUN 88, Glu 116, Mg 2.3, Phos 7.2, Ion Ca 1.13, WBC 19700, H/H 9.7/29.7, Plat 352,000, Segs 51%, Bands 10%, Lymphs 31%, Monos 5%, CRP 43.2

Cultures: Blood: *Staphylococcus epidermidis*

Medication Profile:

Date	Medication
5/21/0300	Folate 1 mg po qd
5/21/0300	MVI 1 po qd
5/21/0300	Iron Sulfate 125 mg po tid
5/21/0300	Epogen 2500 units every 3 weeks
5/21/0300	Oxacillin 900 mg iv q 6 h
5/21/0300	Fortaz 1 gram iv q 8 h

6a. Susan was most likely prescribed iron sulfate because of the concurrent administration of
_____.

A. folate
B. calcium carbonate
C. oxacillin
D. erythropoietin

6b. How many milligrams of elemental iron will Susan receive daily?

A. 75 mg
B. 150 mg
C. 188 mg
D. 375 mg

6c. Which of the following is a potential adverse effect of iron therapy?

   A. Dark stools
   B. Constipation
   C. Stomach irritation
   D. A and B only
   E. A, B, and C

6d. Erythropoietin is primarily produced in the _____.

   A. liver
   B. kidney
   C. muscle
   D. heart

6e. Which of the following routes of administration would be acceptable for Susan's Epogen?

   A. IV
   B. SC
   C. IM
   D. A and B only
   E. A, B, and C

6f. To optimize Susan's Epogen therapy, which of the following parameters are desirable?

   A. Serum ferritin concentration > 100 ng/dL
   B. Transferrin saturation < 20%
   C. Hematocrit > 40%
   D. A and B only
   E. A, B, and C

6g. It may be desirable to interrupt Susan's Epogen therapy if her hematocrit exceeds _____.

   A. 12%
   B. 26%
   C. 30%
   D. 36%

6h. Which of the following is a potential reason for an inadequate response to Epogen therapy?

   A. Iron deficiency
   B. Infection
   C. Inflammation
   D. A and B only
   E. A, B, and C

6i. A potential adverse effect of Epogen therapy in Susan includes _____.

   A. flu-like symptoms
   B. hypertension
   C. seizures
   D. A and B only
   E. A, B, and C

6j. A more appropriate dose of Epogen for Susan would be _____.

   A. 2500 mg every 3 weeks
   B. 2500 mg 3 times per week
   C. 2500 units 3 times per week
   D. 2500 units once per week

6k. Which of the following medications might be considered for Susan?

   A. PhosLo
   B. Calcium acetate
   C. Neutra-Phos K
   D. A and B only
   E. A, B, and C

6l. Which of the following medications is dosed incorrectly for Susan?

   A. Fortaz
   B. Oxacillin
   C. Iron sulfate
   D. A and B only
   E. A, B, and C

6m. Susan's antibiotics were most likely modified because _____.

   A. oxacillin is primarily eliminated via the kidneys and should not be prescribed to patients exhibiting renal dysfunction
   B. ceftazidime is ineffective when prescribed concurrently with vancomycin
   C. the cultured bacteria may have only been sensitive to vancomycin
   D. A and B only

6n. Because of Susan's renal dysfunction, the initial dose of vancomycin should be _____.

   A. as prescribed
   B. as prescribed, but given as two separate doses over the first 12 hours
   C. reduced by 25%
   D. reduced by 50%

6o. Which of the following is the most appropriate strategy in dosing vancomycin in Susan?

   A. As prescribed with vancomycin peak and trough concentrations obtained with third dose
   B. Administer only one dose and obtain a vancomycin concentration in 24 hours
   C. Administer only one dose and obtain two vancomycin concentrations within the first 24–48 hours
   D. As prescribed with vancomycin peak and trough concentrations obtained with the second dose

CASE 7

PHYSICIAN ORDER

Patient Weight: 20 kg

Nifedipine 15 mg sl q 4 h prn
Shohl's solution 15 ml po tid

Date/Time: 03/14/1900
Physician: Glen Morris

Patient Name: Luis Gray
Patient ID #: 213278

MEDICAL PROFILE

Patient: Luis Gray

Patient Weight: 20 kg   **Age:** 8 y/o

Present Illness: Hypertension

Allergies: None

Medical History: Renal disease

Vitals Name: B/P 160/96, P 82, R 14, T 37.5 C

Labs: Na 134, K 4.1, Cl 101, C02 17.3, Cr 3.7, BUN 75, Glu 91, Mg 2.3, Ca 10.8, Phos 8.2, WBC 8500, H/H 11/32, Plat 175,000, Segs 46%, Bands 2%, Lymphs 16%, Monos 4%, CRP 4.3

Medication Profile:

Date	Medication
03/14/1730	Procardia XL 30 mg po qd
03/14/1730	Calcitriol 0.25 mcg qd
03/14/1730	Enalapril 5 mg po bid
03/14/1730	Clonidine 0.1 mg po hs
03/14/1730	Epogen 3000 u qd 3× per week
03/14/1730	Nu-Iron 150 mg po tid
03/14/1730	Folate 1 mg po qd
03/14/1730	MVI 1 po qd
03/14/1730	Calcium carbonate 500 mg po tid
03/14/1730	Furosemide 20 mg iv q 8 h

7a. Which of the following is true regarding Procardia XL?

A. Is classified as an angiotensin-converting enzyme inhibitor

B. May be crushed and administered with tube feedings

C. Contains the same active ingredient as Adalat CC

D. Should initially be dosed twice a day

7b. Calcitriol was prescribed to Luis to _____.

A. promote the intestinal absorption of calcium

B. promote the retention of calcium by the kidneys

C. correct hypercalcemia associated with chronic renal dialysis

D. A and B only

E. A, B, and C

7c. Calcitriol is also known as _____.

   A. 1,25 dihydroxycholecalciferol
   B. Rocaltrol
   C. Calcijex
   D. A and B only
   E. A, B, and C

7d. In the event oral medications were contraindicated in Luis, which of the following might be substituted for his enalapril therapy?

   A. Captopril
   B. Capoten
   C. Enalaprilat
   D. A and B only
   E. A, B, and C

7e. Which of the following is a potential adverse effect from enalapril therapy?

   A. Hypotension
   B. Hyperkalemia
   C. Angioedema
   D. A and B only
   E. A, B, and C

7f. Clonidine is available in which of the following dosage forms?

   A. Tablets
   B. Transdermal patch
   C. Intravenous solution
   D. A and B only
   E. A, B, and C

7g. Clonidine is classified as a(n) _____.

   A. α-antagonist
   B. α- agonist
   C. β- antagonist
   D. β-agonist

7h. Of the following, which is the most likely adverse effect resulting from oral clonidine therapy?

   A. Bradycardia
   B. Insomnia
   C. Excessive salivation
   D. Skin irritation

7i. In the event Luis becomes unable to swallow his clonidine tablet, which of the following would be the most appropriate to prescribe?

   A. Catapres TTS-1
   B. Catapres TTS-2
   C. Catapres TTS-3
   D. Catapres TTS-4

7j. How many mcg/kg/day of clonidine is Luis currently receiving?

   A. 0.5 mcg/kg/day
   B. 1 mcg/kg/day
   C. 5 mcg/kg/day
   D. 10 mcg/kg/day

7k. Which of the following salts contains the most elemental calcium per one gram of the calcium salt?

   A. Calcium chloride
   B. Calcium carbonate
   C. Calcium lactate
   D. Calcium gluconate

7l. Which of the following calcium salts might be more acutely beneficial to Luis?

   A. Calcium gluconate
   B. Calcium chloride
   C. Calcium glubionate
   D. Calcium acetate

7m. How many milligrams per kilogram of elemental calcium is Luis receiving per day?

   A. 7.5 mg/kg
   B. 15 mg/kg
   C. 30 mg/kg
   D. 75 mg/kg

7n. Luis is most likely prescribed Shohl's solution for the treatment of his _____.

   A. hyperphosphatemia
   B. metabolic acidosis
   C. metabolic alkalosis
   D. hypercalcemia

7o. Which of the following is an ingredient found in Shohl's solution?

   A. Sodium citrate
   B. Calcium citrate
   C. Potassium citrate
   D. Magnesium citrate

7p. How many mEq per kilogram of bicarbonate equivalents is Luis receiving per day from his prescribed Shohl's solution?

   A. 1 mEq/kg
   B. 2 mEq/kg
   C. 3 mEq/kg
   D. 4 mEq/kg

7q. Which of the following medications is most similar to nifedipine?

A. Diltiazem
B. Verapamil
C. Nitroprusside
D. Nicardipine

7r. Which of the following is true regarding the most recent nifedipine regimen prescribed to Luis?

A. Is prescribed for its antihypertensive activity
B. Is absorbed rapidly sublingually
C. Should be changed to 10 mg sublingually every 4 hours since it is only available in 10- and 20- mg capsules
D. A and B only
E. A, B, and C

7s. Which of the following is a likely adverse effect from nifedipine?

A. Flushing
B. Bradycardia
C. Atrio-ventricular node block
D. A and B only
E. A, B, and C

7t. Of the following, the most reasonable initial dose of nifedipine for Luis would be _____.

A. as prescribed
B. 2 mg
C. 5 mg
D. 10 mg

CASE 8

PHYSICIAN ORDER

Patient Weight: <u>40 kg</u>

Potassium chloride 20 mEq po bid
Propranolol 5 mg po q 6 h

Date/Time: <u>11/12/0900</u>
Physician: <u>Bret Baker</u>

Patient Name: <u>Jerry Tessler</u>
Patient ID #: <u>789098</u>

MEDICAL PROFILE

Patient: Jerry Tessler

Patient Weight: 40 kg   **Age:** 7 y/o

Present Illness: Trauma, hypertension, transferred to floor from ICU

Allergies: None

Medical History: Asthma, urinary stones

Labs: Na 132, K 3.2, Cl 96, C02 27, Cr 0.6, BUN 7, Glu 114, Mg 1.9, Ca 10.3, WBC 4600, H/H 12.4/37.2, Plat 157,000, Segs 62%, Bands 2%, Lymphs 3%, Monos 1%

Vitals Name: B/P 130/77, P 84, R 12, T 37 C

Medication Profile:

Date	Medication
11/11/2100	Furosemide 20 mg po bid
11/11/2100	Metolazone 5 mg po qd
11/11/2100	Cefazolin 1 gm iv q 8 h
11/11/2100	Fluticasone 1 puff q 12 h
11/11/2100	Albuterol 1–2 puffs q 4–6 h prn

8a. Which of the following is a potential cause of secondary hypertension in pediatric patients?

A. Acute nephritis
B. Increased intracranial pressure
C. Seizures
D. A and B only
E. A, B, and C

8b. Furosemide is classified as a(n) _____ diuretic.

A. loop
B. thiazide
C. potassium-sparing
D. osmotic

8c. Which of the following is a potential adverse effect of furosemide therapy?

   A. Hypokalemia
   B. Hypochloremic metabolic alkalosis
   C. Hypercalciuria
   D. A and B only
   E. A, B, and C

8d. Which of the following is most similar to furosemide?

   A. Bumetanide
   B. Hydrochlorothiazide
   C. Metolazone
   D. Amiloride

8e. The equivalent intravenous dose of furosemide for Jerry is _____ mg.

   A. 5
   B. 7.5
   C. 10
   D. 20

8f. Given Jerry's medical history, which of the following diuretics might be better tolerated?

   A. Ethacrynic acid
   B. Torsemide
   C. Bumetanide
   D. Chlorothiazide

8g. Metolazone is most closely related to _____.

   A. hydrochlorothiazide
   B. furosemide
   C. acetazolamide
   D. spironolactone

8h. What is the rationale for prescribing both furosemide and metolazone to Jerry?

   A. Both act at similar nephron sites resulting in increased diuresis
   B. Both act at different nephron sites resulting in increased diuresis
   C. Combined therapy results in decreased electrolyte loss
   D. Combined therapy results in less glucose intolerance

8i. Which of the following would most likely pose a problem if prescribed concurrently with Jerry's potassium chloride?

   A. Amiloride
   B. Triamterene
   C. Spironolactone
   D. A and B only
   E. A, B, and C

8j. Which of the following is true of Jerry's potassium-chloride therapy?

   A. May result in gastrointestinal adverse effects
   B. Should be administered intravenously to decrease risk of adverse effects
   C. Should be administered undiluted for maximal efficacy
   D. For optimal response, once daily dosing should be encouraged

8k. Propranolol is classified as a(n) _____.

   A. calcium channel antagonist
   B. β-adrenergic antagonist
   C. angiotensin-receptor blocker
   D. angiotensin-converting enzyme inhibitor

8l. Adverse effects associated with propranolol include _____.

   A. tachycardia
   B. bronchodilation
   C. CNS stimulation
   D. decreased libido

8m. Propranolol is available in which of the following dosage forms?

   A. Tablets
   B. Sustained-released capsules
   C. Injection
   D. A and B only
   E. A, B, and C

8n. In lieu of propranolol, which of the following would be more appropriate to prescribe to Jerry?

   A. Atenolol
   B. Nadolol
   C. Timolol
   D. Sotalol

80. Which of the following is the most significant difference between propranolol and labetalol?

    A. Labetalol is selective for β-1 receptors
    B. Labetalol antagonizes α-1 receptors
    C. Labetalol is only available as an injectable solution
    D. Labetalol is not indicated for the treatment of hypertension

CASE 9

PHYSICIAN ORDER

Patient Weight: 30 kg

Morphine sulfate 3 mg iv q 2–3 h prn
Clindamycin 400 mg iv q 6 h

Date/Time: 6/15/0900
Physician: Ray Burrows

Patient Name: Linda London
Patient ID #: 213278

MEDICAL PROFILE

Patient: Linda London

Patient Weight: 30 kg **Age:** 7 y/o

Present Illness: Appendicitis

Allergies: None

Medical History: Unremarkable

Labs: Na 136, K 3.6, Cl 105, C02 23.9, Cr 0.6, BUN 5, Glu 103, WBC 16100, H/H 14.6/42.2, Plat 260,000, Segs 84%, Bands 4%, Lymphs 5%, Monos 7%, gentamicin 25 mcg/ml on 6/14 at 1100

Medication Profile:

Date	Medication
6/14/0900	Gentamicin 225 mg iv qd
6/14/0900	Acetaminophen with codeine 1 tsp po q 4 h prn

9a. Which of the following is true regarding appendicitis?

  A. Is the least common condition requiring emergency surgery in children
  B. Occurs most commonly in males and peaks at 30 to 40 years of age
  C. Sudden diminution of pain indicates acute remission
  D. Is more difficult to diagnose in adolescent females than in males

9b. The gentamicin was prescribed to Linda for its coverage against _____.

  A. gram-positive bacteria
  B. gram-negative bacteria
  C. anaerobes
  D. atypical bacteria

9c. Which of the following best describes gentamicin's antibacterial activity?

  A. Concentration-dependent bactericidal activity
  B. Concentration-dependent bacteriostatic activity
  C. Concentration-independent bactericidal activity
  D. Concentration-independent bacteriostatic activity

9d. Linda's gentamicin was administered at 10:00 am on June 14th as a 30-minute infusion. Which of the following is true of the reported gentamicin concentration?

  A. It represents a peak concentration
  B. It represents a trough concentration
  C. The concentration is excessive and therefore the dose will need to be decreased
  D. The concentration was obtained on the first dose and therefore is invalid
  E. A and C only

9e.   Linda's gentamicin trough concentration is reported as undetectable. This most likely indicates that _____.

    A.   the dosing interval is too long
    B.   bacterial resistance is most likely to occur
    C.   the dosing interval is adequate
    D.   her kidney function is compromised

9f.   Which of the following is associated with gentamicin?

    A.   Penicillin-binding proteins
    B.   Postantibiotic effect
    C.   50-S ribosomal binding
    D.   DNA gyrase activity

9g.   Which of the following adverse effects is most commonly mentioned with respect to gentamicin therapy?

    A.   Bone marrow suppression
    B.   Hepatic toxicity
    C.   Seizures
    D.   Renal insufficiency

9h.   Which of the following would have been the most appropriate alternative gentamicin regimen to prescribe to Linda?

    A.   30 mg iv q 8 h
    B.   60 mg iv q 12 h
    C.   75 mg iv q 8 h
    D.   90 mg iv q 8 h

9i.   Which of the following medications is most closely related to gentamicin?

    A.   Clindamycin
    B.   Tobramycin
    C.   Cefotaxime
    D.   Piperacillin

9j.   How many milligrams of codeine will Linda receive with each dose of her acetaminophen-with-codeine preparation?

    A.   5 mg
    B.   12 mg
    C.   15 mg
    D.   22 mg

9k.   Clindamycin is classified as a _____.

    A.   penicillin
    B.   lincosamide
    C.   cephalosporin
    D.   glycopeptide

9l.   The trade name for clindamycin is _____.

    A.   Cloxapen
    B.   Biaxin
    C.   Cleocin
    D.   Claforan

9m.   Clindamycin was most likely prescribed for Linda because of its activity against _____.

    A.   gram-positive bacteria
    B.   gram-negative bacteria
    C.   anaerobes
    D.   atypicals

9n.   Which of the following is most often associated with clindamycin therapy?

    A.   Renal dysfunction
    B.   Pseudomembranous colitis
    C.   Seizures
    D.   Ototoxicity

9o.   Clindamycin is available is which of the following dosage forms?

    A.   Capsules
    B.   Lotion
    C.   Cream
    D.   B and C only
    E.   A, B, and C

9p.   Which of the following is most closely related to clindamycin?

    A.   Lincomycin
    B.   Azithromycin
    C.   Clonazepam
    D.   Cefepime

9q.   Which of the following is true regarding the administration of Linda's clindamycin?

    A.   May be combined with gentamicin in the same intravenous bag
    B.   Should be infused at least 1 hour after her gentamicin infusion
    C.   Should be infused at least 1 hour before her gentamicin infusion
    D.   Should be protected from light during administration

9r. Clindamycin is available as a 150 mg/mL intravenous preparation. How many milliliters are needed to provide Linda with her prescribed dose?

A. 1.3 mL
B. 2.7 mL
C. 3.4 mL
D. 5.2 mL

9s. Which of the following would be a more appropriate clindamycin regimen for Linda?

A. 400 mg iv q 8 h
B. 400 mg iv q 12 h
C. 600 mg iv q 8 h
D. 600 mg iv q 12 h

9t. Which of the following is the most likely reason intravenous morphine is prescribed for Linda?

A. Codeine for injection is not available
B. Administering morphine will likely result in less complaints of itching
C. Is intended to be available if Linda experiences moderate to severe pain
D. B and C only
E. A, B, and C

CASE 10

PHYSICIAN ORDER

Patient Weight: <u>30 kg</u>

Metronidazole 500 mg iv q 8 h
Ampicillin 1500 mg iv q 12 h

Date/Time: <u>07/05/1700</u>
Physician: <u>John Hughes</u>

Patient Name: <u>Lisa Moore</u>
Patient ID #: <u>217878</u>

MEDICAL PROFILE

Patient: Lisa Moore

Patient Weight: 30 kg   **Age:** 7 y/o

Present Illness: Gastroenteritis

Allergies: None

Medical History: Unremarkable

Labs: Na 138, K 4.7, Cl 101, C02 22, Cr 0.5, BUN 6, Glu 89, Mg 2.1, WBC 8500, H/H 13/39.1, Plat 242,000, Segs 46%, Bands 17%, Lymphs 26%, Monos 10%, CRP 7.2, Alk Phos 62, AST 16, ALT 12, T Bili 0.5, D Bili 0.0, I Bili 0.5, Total Prot 7.5, Alb 3.9

Cultures: Pending

Medication Profile:

Date	Medication
7/5/0800	Ranitidine 30 mg iv q 8 h
7/5/0800	Carafate 500 mg iv q 6 h
7/5/0800	Acetaminophen 450 mg po q 6 h prn

10a. Which of the following is the generic name for Carafate?

A. Famotidine
B. Nizatidine
C. Sucralfate
D. Ranitidine

10b. Which of the following best describes the mechanism of action of Carafate?

A. Histamine antagonist
B. Proton-pump inhibitor
C. Prokinetic agent
D. Mucosal protectant

10c. Carafate should be used with caution in patients with renal failure because it contains _____.

A. magnesium
B. aluminum
C. sodium
D. phosphorus

10d. Lisa's Carafate regimen should be modified to _____.

A. 500 mg iv q 8 h
B. 500 mg po q 6 h
C. 1 gram iv q 6 h
D. 1 gram po q 6 h

10e. The trade name for metronidazole is _____.

    A. Flagyl
    B. Floxin
    C. Zyban
    D. Zyprexa

10f. Lisa is prescribed metronidazole because of its activity against _____.

    A. gram-positive bacteria
    B. gram-negative bacteria
    C. anaerobic bacteria
    D. A and C only
    E. A, B, and C

10g. Metronidazole is prescribed for peptic ulcer disease because of its activity against _____.

    A. *Helicobacter pylori*
    B. *Salmonella*
    C. *Streptococcus pyogenes*
    D. *Streptococcus pneumoniae*

10h. Which of the following adverse effects is most closely associated with metronidazole?

    A. Peripheral neuropathy
    B. Optic neuritis
    C. Renal dysfunction
    D. Ototoxicity

10i. Alcoholic beverages should not be consumed by a patient receiving metronidazole therapy because of the possibility of _____ occurring.

    A. the production of nephrotoxic substances
    B. a disulfiram-type reaction
    C. a Steven Johnson-like syndrome
    D. Reye's syndrome

10j. Which of the following is true of neutralized metronidazole solutions for injection?

    A. Should be stored under refrigeration until administered
    B. Should be protected from light
    C. Is available in 10 mg/mL ready to use containers
    D. A and B only
    E. A, B, and C

10k. Which of Lisa's laboratory values warrants close monitoring during her metronidazole therapy?

    A. Serum creatinine
    B. White blood cell count
    C. Sodium
    D. Magnesium

10l. Which of the following would be a more appropriate metronidazole regimen for Lisa?

    A. 225 mg iv q 6 h
    B. 500 mg iv q 6 h
    C. 750 mg iv q 8 h
    D. 1 gram iv q 6 h

10m. Which of the following bacteria would most likely be eradicated by ampicillin therapy?

    A. *Listeria*
    B. *Mycoplasma*
    C. *Pseudomonas*
    D. *Bacteroides*

10n. Which of the following is true regarding ampicillin for intravenous use?

    A. Reconstituted solution is stable for 24 hours
    B. Dextrose is the preferred diluent for the reconstituted solutions
    C. May also be administered intramuscularly
    D. A and B only
    E. A, B, and C

10o. A more appropriate ampicillin regimen for Lisa would be _____.

    A. 1 gram iv q 8 h
    B. 1 gram iv q 6 h
    C. 1500 mg iv q 8 h
    D. 2000 gm iv q 8 h

CASE 11

PHYSICIAN ORDER

Patient Weight: 20 kg

PZA 600 mg po qd
Acetaminophen 300 mg po q 6 h prn

Date/Time: 10/19/1400
Physician: Bill Tucker

Patient Name: Robert Gordon
Patient ID #: 963278

MEDICAL PROFILE

Patient: Robert Gordon

Patient Weight: 20 kg   **Age:** 5 y/o

Present Illness: TB

Allergies: None

Medical History: Asthma

Labs: Na 138, K 3.7, Cl 111, C02 23, Cr 0.3, BUN 4, Glu 102, Mg 2.2, Ion Ca 1.11, WBC 14,000, H/H 11.3/34.1, Plat 175,000, Segs 48%, Bands 7%, Lymphs 15%, Monos 4%, Alk Phos 73, ALT 13, AST 23, T Bili 1, D Bili 0.4, I Bili 0.6, Total Protein 6.5, Alb 3.5, CRP 11, Theophylline 13.5

Tests/Cultures: PPD placed and sputum gram stain pending

Medication Profile:

Date	Medication
10/19/0900	Rifampin 300 mg po qd
10/19/0900	INH 300 mg po qid
10/19/0900	Albuterol 2.5 mg neb q 3 h prn
10/19/0900	Flovent 1 puff q 12 h
10/19/0900	Aminophylline 20 mg/hr

11a. Which of the following is true regarding tuberculosis?

   A. Is caused by the pathogen *Mycobacterium tuberculosis*
   B. Is primarily transmitted from person-to-person via an oral/fecal route
   C. Most strains of the offending pathogen are rapidly growing
   D. A and C only
   E. A, B, and C

11b. Because of their staining properties, the bacteria associated with tuberculosis are referred to as

_____.

   A. aerobic cocci
   B. aerobic bacilli
   C. acid fast bacilli
   D. anaerobic cocci

11c. The PPD test placed on Robert refers to a _____ test.

  A. plasma-protein derivative
  B. purified-protein derivative
  C. polyvalent-peptide disc
  D. pulmonary-peptide disc

11d. Which of the following is true of the PPD test?

  A. A 5-tuberculin unit dose is most often used
  B. The test should be read within 48–72 hours
  C. Tubersol is the preferred marketed product
  D. A and B only
  E. A, B, and C

11e. Which of the following medications is typically the primary treatment for latent tuberculosis?

  A. Rifampin
  B. INH
  C. PZA
  D. Ethambutol

11f. The addition of PZA to Robert's regimen will likely reduce his tuberculosis treatment course to _____ months.

  A. 3
  B. 6
  C. 9
  D. 12

11g. Which of the following adverse effects is associated with PZA therapy?

  A. Hyperuricemia
  B. Gastrointestinal distress
  C. Hepatotoxicity
  D. A and B only
  E. A, B, and C

11h. The concurrent administration of which of the following of Robert's medications might necessitate an aminophylline dosing change?

  A. Flovent
  B. PZA
  C. Rifampin
  D. Albuterol

11i. INH is a synonym for _____.

  A. isoniazid
  B. isonicotinic-acid hydrazide
  C. isonicotinic-acid hydrochloride
  D. A and B only
  E. A and C only

11j. Which of the following vitamins would be most appropriate to prescribe to Robert?

  A. B1
  B. B3
  C. B6
  D. B12

11k. Which of the following adverse events is most closely associated with INH therapy?

  A. Optic neuritis
  B. Nephrotoxicity
  C. Arrhythmias
  D. Peripheral neuropathy

11l. Which of the following would be a more appropriate INH regimen for Robert?

  A. 150 mg po qd
  B. 300 mg po qd
  C. 300 mg po bid
  D. 300 mg po tid

11m. Rifampin is bactericidal against which of the following organisms?

  A. *Mycobacterium bovis*
  B. *Mycobacterium kansasii*
  C. *Mycobacterium avium* complex
  D. A and B only
  E. A, B, and C

11n. Which of the following is true of rifampin therapy?

  A. May only be administered orally
  B. Is an inhibitor of the cytochrome P450 isoenzyme system
  C. May result in red-orange discoloration of bodily secretions
  D. B and C only
  E. A, B, and C

11o. Which of the following in the major adverse effect associated with ethambutol therapy?

  A. Hepatotoxicity
  B. Retrobulbar neuritis
  C. Nephrotoxicity
  D. Seizures

CASE 12

PHYSICIAN ORDER

Patient Weight: 50 kg

Amphotericin B Liposomal 50 mg iv qd

Date/Time: 11/05/1100
Physician: Jeff Boyles

Patient Name: Leonard Newell
Patient ID #: 785693

MEDICAL PROFILE

Patient: Leonard Newell

Patient Weight: 50 kg   **Age:** 16 y/o

Present Illness: AML

Allergies: None

Medical History: S/P treatment with Ara-C and daunorubicin

Labs: Na 135, K 3.3, Cl 105, C02 26.1, Cr 0.4, BUN 8, Glu 160, Mg 1.6, WBC 300, H/H 7.6/21.4, Plat 26,000, Segs 0%, Bands 0%, Lymphs 10%, Monos 0%,CRP 8, Alk Phos 78, AST 10, ALT 12, T Bili 1.2, D Bili 0.5, I Bili 0.7, Total Prot 5.4, Alb 2.9, Phos 4.7, Mg 1.7.

Cultures: Pending

Medication Profile:

Date	Medication
11/5/0700	Ranitidine 50 mg iv q 8 h
11/5/0700	Zofran 8 mg iv q 8 h prn
11/5/0700	Peridex prn
11/5/0700	Morphine sulfate PCA per protocol
11/5/0700	Narcan 0.4 mg iv prn
11/5/0700	Benadryl 25 mg iv q 4–6 h prn
11/5/0700	Vancomycin 1 gm iv q 8 h
11/5/0700	Fortaz 2 gm iv q 8 h
11/5/0700	Colace 100 mg po hs

12a. Which of the following is a synonym for Ara-C?

A. Cytarabine hydrochloride
B. Cytosine-Arabinosine hydrochloride
C. CytoGam
D. A and B only
E. A, B, and C

12b. Which of the following is true regarding Ara-C?

A. Is converted intracellularly to cytarabine triphosphate
B. Mechanism of action involves inhibition of miotic spindle formation
C. Readily penetrates the blood-brain barrier
D. May only be administered via intravenous infusion

12c. Which of the following is a major toxicity associated with Ara-C?

A. Myelosuppression
B. Alopecia
C. Hepatotoxicity
D. A and B only
E. A, B, and C

12d. Which of the following best describes the mechanism of action of daunorubicin?

A. Binds DNA-preventing transcription
B. Acts as an alkylating agent to inhibit DNA synthesis
C. Inhibits miotic spindle formation
D. Inhibits DNA and RNA synthesis by DNA intercalation

12e. Which of the following is the major toxicity associated with daunorubicin therapy?

A. Neurotoxicity
B. Pulmonary fibrosis
C. Cardiotoxicity
D. Nephrotoxicity

12f. Which of the following is true of daunorubicin?

A. Transient red-orange discoloration of the urine may occur
B. May be administered intravenously or intramuscularly
C. Is metabolized to an active metabolite, daunorubicinol
D. A and C only
E. A, B, and C

12g. Which of the following medications is most similar to daunorubicin?

A. Adriamycin
B. 5-FU
C. Cisplatin
D. Asparaginase

12h. Which of the following medications may have been prescribed to Leonard to prevent acute urate nephropathy induced by his chemotherapy regimen?

A. Ifosfamide
B. Ibuprofen
C. MESNA
D. Allopurinol

12i. The most likely reason for prescribing diphenhydramine to Leonard was to _____.

A. treat itching that might result from morphine therapy
B. prevent the occurrence of a rash that is likely to occur with vancomycin
C. enhance the effects of ranitidine
D. counter the effects of naloxone in the event toxicity develops

12j. Which of the following is the most likely reason for prescribing ceftazidime and vancomycin to Leonard?

A. Broad-spectrum antibiotic coverage in the presence of neutropenia
B. Provide coverage for *Staphylococcal* infections in the presence of thrombocytopenia
C. Synergistic activity against *Pseudomonas*
D. Prevent resistance for *Staphylococcal* infections

12k. Pending serum concentrations, the dose of vancomycin for Leonard should be

_____.

A. increased to 1 gm iv q 6 h
B. decreased to 500 mg iv q 6 h
C. decreased to 500 mg iv q 8 h
D. unaltered

12l. Which of Leonard's lab values necessitates close monitoring with his newly prescribed antifungal therapy?

A. Sodium
B. Potassium
C. Magnesium
D. B and C only
E. A, B, and C

12m. Which of the following is the most appropriate indication for a "lipid" formulation of amphotericin B?

A. Empiric therapy for systemic fungal infections
B. Patients refractory to conventional amphotericin-B therapy
C. Patients with hepatic dysfunction
D. Fungal infection involving the central nervous system

12n. Typically, the dose-limiting adverse effect of amphotericin-B therapy is _____.

A. Nephrotoxicity
B. Neurotoxicity
C. Myelosuppression
D. Rigors

12o. Which of the following best describes the mechanism of action of Leonard's antifungal therapy?

    A. Binding to the fungal 30s ribosome thus inhibiting protein synthesis

    B. Interacting with fungal DNA gyrase thus inhibiting protein synthesis

    C. Binding to sterols in fungal cell wall

    D. Interacting with peptidoglycans in fungal cell wall

12p. Administering _____ may decrease the duration of the shaking chills associated with amphotericin-B therapy.

    A. meperidine

    B. promethazine

    C. hydrocortisone

    D. acetaminophen

12q. Given the physician's antifungal medication order, which of the following products should be dispensed to Leonard?

    A. Fungizone

    B. Amphotec

    C. Abelcet

    D. Ambisone

12r. A more appropriate dose of amphotericin-B liposomal for Leonard would be _____ .

    A. 100 mg iv qd

    B. 100 mg iv q 12 h

    C. 200 mg iv qd

    D. 300 mg iv qd

CASE 13

PHYSICIAN ORDER

Patient Weight: <u>24 kg</u>

Vincristine 1 mg iv
Asparaginase 5500 IU
Prednisone 35 mg po qd

Date/Time: <u>05/21/0900</u>
Physician: <u>Sam Perks</u>

Patient Name: <u>Ben Jones</u>
Patient ID #: <u>367878</u>

MEDICAL PROFILE

Patient: Ben Jones

Patient Weight: 24 kg   **Age:** 4 y/o

BSA: 0.9 m^2

Present Illness: ALL

Allergies: None

Medical History: Bruises easily, anorexia, malaise, intermittent fever

Labs: Na 136, K 3.6, Cl 106, C02 22, Cr 0.4, BUN 9, Glu 124, Mg 1.9, WBC 6000, H/H 10.8/31.6, Plat 60,000, Segs 58%, Bands 1%, Lymphs 32%, Monos 10%, CRP 4, Alk Phos 74, AST 24, ALT 16, T Bili 0.6, D Bili 0.1, I Bili 0.5, Total Prot 5.3, Alb 3.5

Cultures: Pending

Medication Profile:

Date	Medication
5/20/1800	Ranitidine 25 mg iv q 8 h
5/20/1800	Zofran 3.5 mg iv q 8 h prn
5/20/1800	Peridex prn
5/20/1800	Morphine sulfate 0.12 mg iv q 2–3 h prn pain
5/20/1800	Narcan iv prn
5/20/1800	Benadryl 25 mg iv q 6 h prn
5/20/1800	Allopurinol 100 mg po tid

13a.   Which of the following statements is true regarding ALL?

  A. Diagnosis at an age of older than 1 year or younger than 15 years is associated with a poor prognosis
  B. The leukemic cells of children with ALL are usually quite resistant to chemotherapy
  C. The bone marrow of ALL patients is usually completely replaced with leukemic lymphoblasts
  D. Initially, the platelet counts of ALL patients are usually normal to extremely high

13b.   Which of the following is a likely consequence of Ben's morphine therapy?

  A. Constipation
  B. Tolerance
  C. Psychological addiction
  D. A and B only
  E. A, B, and C

13c.   A more appropriate initial morphine dose for Ben would be _____.

  A. 1.2 mg
  B. 1.2 mcg
  C. 4.8 mg
  D. 4.8 mcg

13d.   Which of the following actions would be most appropriate in the event Ben is requiring doses of morphine every 2–3 hours for pain relief?

  A. Maintain the same dose, but administer every 1 hour
  B. Increase the dose, but maintain the same prn schedule
  C. Increase the dose and establish a scheduled dosing interval
  D. Maintain the same dose, but place the patient on a PCA pump

13e.   Which of the following is the most likely reason for prescribing naloxone to Ben?

  A. Used as an antidote in the event toxicity results from morphine therapy
  B. To rapidly reverse the effects of morphine once analgesic therapy is discontinued
  C. To prolong the analgesic effects of morphine
  D. Used to treat pruritus that often results from morphine therapy

13f.   An appropriate dose of naloxone for Ben would be _____.

  A. 0.024 mg
  B. 0.24 mg
  C. 0.04 mg
  D. 0.4 mg

13g.   The trade name for vincristine is _____.

  A. Velban
  B. Velsar
  C. Oncovin
  D. Omnipen

13h.   Which of the following best describes the mechanism of action of vincristine?

  A. Alkylating agent
  B. Inhibitor of DNA polymerase
  C. Inhibitor of miotic-spindle formation
  D. Inhibits purine biosynthesis

13i.   Which of the following adverse effects is associated with vincristine therapy?

  A. Alopecia
  B. Neurotoxicity
  C. Inappropriate ADH secretion
  D. A and B only
  E. A, B, and C

13j.   Ben's vincristine should be dosed _____.

  A. once a day
  B. twice a day
  C. once a week
  D. once a month

13k.   The maximum recommended single dose of vincristine is _____ mg.

  A. 1
  B. 2
  C. 3
  D. 4

13l.   The recommended route(s) of administration of vincristine is(are) _____.

  A. intravenous
  B. intrathecal
  C. intramuscular
  D. A and B only
  E. A, B, and C

13m. The trade name for asparaginase is _____.

    A. Elspar
    B. Atacand
    C. Paraplatin
    D. Oncaspar

13n. Which of the following adverse effects is most commonly associated with asparaginase therapy?

    A. Anorexia
    B. Convulsions
    C. Pancreatitis
    D. Local allergic reactions

13o. Ben's asparaginase dose should be administered _____.

    A. once daily
    B. three times a week
    C. once weekly
    D. once monthly

13p. The preferred administration route for Ben's asparaginase therapy is _____.

    A. intravenous
    B. intramuscular
    C. intrathecal
    D. subcutaneous

13q. Asparaginase is available as 10,000 units per vial and is reconstituted in 2 mL of normal saline. How many milliliters of the resultant solution are needed to provide Ben with his prescribed dose?

    A. 0.55 mL
    B. 1.1 mL
    C. 1.8 mL
    D. 2.2 mL

13r. Ben will most likely receive prednisone therapy for _____ days.

    A. 3
    B. 5
    C. 15
    D. 28

13s. Which of the following adverse effects might Ben encounter as a result of his prednisone therapy?

    A. Adrenal suppression
    B. Hyperglycemia
    C. Gastrointestinal disturbances
    D. A and C only
    E. A, B, and C

13t. Which of the following medications would likely be considered as an additional treatment of Ben's ALL?

    A. Methotrexate
    B. Etoposide
    C. Cisplatin
    D. Cyclophosphamide

CASE 14

PHYSICIAN ORDER

Patient Weight: 50 kg

Cyclophosphamide 1125 mg iv on day 1
Doxorubicin 75 mg on day 1
Vincristine 2 mg iv on day 1 and 5
Prednisone 150 mg/day on days 1–5

Date/Time: 07/15/0900
Physician: Everett Jacobs

Patient Name: Heather Walker
Patient ID #: 215478

MEDICAL PROFILE

Patient: Heather Walker

Present Illness: Non-Hodgkin's lymphoma

Medical History: Unremarkable

Patient Weight: 50 kg   **Age:** 16 y/o

BSA: 1.5 m²

Allergies: None

Labs: Na 136, K 3.9, Cl 109, C02 20, Cr 0.4, BUN 7, Glu 110, Mg 2.3, WBC 6500, H/H 12/36.1, Plat 250,000, Segs 55%, Bands 5%, Lymphs 32%, Monos 10%, CRP 3, Alk Phos 56, AST 24, ALT 32, T Bili 0.4, D Bili 0.0, I Bili 0.4, Total Prot 5.5, Alb 4.1

Cultures: Pending

Medication Profile:

Date	Medication
7/14/2100	Allopurinol 300 mg po tid
7/14/2100	Ranitidine 50 mg iv q 8 h
7/14/2100	Zofran 8 mg iv prior to cyclophosphamide and q 8 h prn
7/14/2100	Morphine sulfate 5mg iv q 2–4 hours as needed
7/14/2100	Diphenhydramine 25 mg iv q 6 h prn
7/14/2100	Peridex prn

14a. The acronym for the chemotherapy regimen prescribed for Heather is _____.

A. CDVP
B. PVDC
C. POCR
D. CHOP

14b. The trade name for cyclophosphamide is _____.

A. Cytosar
B. Cytoxan
C. Cytomel
D. Cytovene

14c. Which of the following best categorizes the therapeutic activity of cyclophosphamide?

   A. Miotic-spindle inhibitor
   B. Alkylating agent
   C. DNA-polymerase inhibitor
   D. Pyrimidine-synthesis inhibitor

14d. Which of the following adverse effects is commonly associated with cyclophosphamide therapy?

   A. Alopecia
   B. Myelosuppression
   C. Metallic taste
   D. A and B only
   E. A, B, and C

14e. Which of the following is true regarding the administration of cyclophosphamide?

   A. Aggressive hydration is recommended
   B. Recommended minimal concentration of the reconstituted solution is 50 mg/mL
   C. Is only available for intravenous use
   D. As a result of extended infusion times, diluents containing preservatives are recommended

14f. Which of the following drugs may be prescribed to Heather to prevent cyclophosphamide-induced hemorrhagic cystitis?

   A. Ifosfamide
   B. Mesna
   C. Thioguanine
   D. Mycophenolate

14g. The trade name for doxorubicin is _____.

   A. Adriamycin
   B. Zinecard
   C. Doryx
   D. Adrucil

14h. Which of the following is a potential adverse effect of doxorubicin therapy?

   A. Myelosuppression
   B. Alopecia
   C. Pink or red urine color
   D. A and B only
   E. A, B, and C

14i. Heather's doxorubicin dose should be administered _____.

   A. orally
   B. intramuscularly
   C. subcutaneously
   D. intravenously

14j. Because of the potential of irreversible cardiotoxicity, the maximum recommended total dose of doxorubicin is _____ mg/m^2.

   A. 250
   B. 350
   C. 450
   D. 550

14k. Heather is subsequently prescribed G-CSF 300 mg sc bid. The G-CSF is intended to resolve her _____.

   A. anemia
   B. neutropenia
   C. thrombocytopenia
   D. pancytopenia

14l. G-CSF is also known as _____.

   A. Neupogen
   B. Prokine
   C. Epogen
   D. A and B only
   E. A, B, and C

14m. Which of the following is true regarding the administration of G-CSF?

   A. Is typically given within 24 hours following the administration of chemotherapy
   B. An increase in cell counts may be seen within 1–2 days of initiation of therapy
   C. May only be administered subcutaneously
   D. Is contraindicated in patients with a documented allergy to penicillin

14n. Which of the following adverse effects is associated with G-CSF therapy?

   A. Bone pain
   B. Arthralgia
   C. Fever
   D. B and C only
   E. A, B, and C

14o. A more appropriate G-CSF regimen for Heather would be _____.

   A. 150 mcg sc bid
   B. 150 mg sc qd
   C. 300 mg sc qd
   D. 300 mcg sc qd

CASE 15

PERIPHERAL TPN ORDER

Patient Name: Lewis Burgess
Patient ID# 896598

Patient Weight: 20 kg

Amino Acid: 2%
Dextrose: 10%

Additives:

NaCl 6 mEq/L
Na Acetate 24 mEq/L
KCL 6 mEq/L
K Phosphate 14 mEq/L

Mg Sulfate 4.16 mEq/L
Ca Gluconate 20 mEq/L
PTE-5 2 mLs
MVI Pediatric 5 mLs

TPN Infusion Rate: 55 mLs/hr over 24 hours

Intravenous Fats 20%: 17 mLs/hr over 12 hours

Date/Time: 01/24/1100

Physician: David Smyth

MEDICAL PROFILE

Patient: Lewis Burgess

Present Illness: R/O Pancreatitis

Patient Weight: 20 kg   **Age:** 5 y/o

Allergies: None

Medical History: Unremarkable

Labs: Na 133, K 3.8, Cl 101, C02 32, Cr 0.6, BUN 4, Glu 91, Mg 2.1, ICA 1.13, Phos 3.6, WBC 4500, H/H 12/36.1, Plat 242,000, Segs 46%, Bands 5%, Lymphs 10%, Monos 3%, Alk Phos 64, AST 10, ALT 15, T Bili 0.5, D Bili 0.0, Total Prot 7.1, Alb 2.4

Cultures: Pending

Medication Profile:

Date	Medication
1/23/2100	Meperidine 20 mg iv q 2–4 h prn pain

15a. Obtaining which of the following lab values would be most helpful in determining a diagnosis for Lewis?

A. Arterial blood gas
B. Prothrombin time
C. C-reactive protein
D. Amylase

15b. Which of the following is the most likely reason for prescribing meperidine in lieu of morphine for Lewis?

A. Meperidine is a more potent opiate
B. Meperidine has less potential to induce seizure activity
C. Morphine is believed to have more adverse effects on the sphincter of oddi
D. Tolerance develops more commonly with morphine

15c. Which of the following would be a more appropriate analgesic regimen for Lewis?

A. Meperidine 2 mg iv q 2–4 h prn
B. Meperidine 4 mg iv q 2–4 h prn
C. Morphine 2 mg iv q 2–4 h prn
D. Morphine 5 mg iv q 2–4 h prn

15d. Of the following lab values, which would be most appropriate to obtain for Lewis?

A. L-cysteine
B. Triglycerides
C. Indirect bilirubin
D. Procalcitonin

15e. The recommended caloric requirement for Lewis is approximately _____ kcal/kg/day.

A. 30–60
B. 75–90
C. 85–130
D. 90–100

15f. Which of the following is true of the type of TPN prescribed for Lewis?

A. May require large volumes to meet nutritional requirements
B. Risk of phlebitis is increased when simultaneously infusing lipids with the amino acid/dextrose solution
C. Infections are the most common complication
D. A and B only
E. A, B, and C

15g. Which of the following is the most common metabolic complication resulting from TPN administration?

A. Hyperphosphatemia
B. Hyperglycemia
C. Hypokalemia
D. Hypomagnesemia

15h. Which of the following amino acid solutions would most likely be used for Lewis' TPN?

A. Travasol
B. TrophAmine
C. HepatAmine
D. NephrAmine

15i. The osmolarity of the dextrose solution prescribed for Lewis is _____ mOsm/L.

A. 250
B. 500
C. 750
D. 1000

15j. The dextrose component of Lewis' TPN provides him with _____ kilocalories per day.

A. 250
B. 350
C. 450
D. 550

15k. Approximately how many milliliters of a 70% dextrose solution are needed to prepare Lewis' TPN?

A. 70 mL
B. 100 mL
C. 150 mL
D. 190 mL

15l. Typically, the maximum recommended concentration of dextrose for Lewis' TPN is _____ %.

A. 10
B. 12.5
C. 15
D. 20

15m. The intravenous fat regimen prescribed for Lewis provides him with approximately _____ kilo-calories.

A. 200
B. 250
C. 400
D. 450

15n. Approximately how many milliequivalents of sodium will Lewis receive daily via his TPN?

A. 24 mEq
B. 30 mEq
C. 40 mEq
D. 50 mEq

15o. Lewis is receiving 14 mEq/L of potassium as potassium phosphate. Approximately how many millimoles of phosphorus is he receiving per day from this potassium-phosphate preparation?

A. 13 mMol
B. 15 mMol
C. 17 mMol
D. 19 mMol

15p. Of the following additives, which one would most likely be omitted from Lewis' TPN?

A. Ca Gluconate
B. Na Acetate
C. Mg Sulfate
D. K Phosphate

15q. Which of following is a component of PTE-5?

A. Chromium
B. Copper
C. L-cysteine
D. A and B only
E. A, B, and C

CASE 16

CENTRAL TPN ORDER

Patient Name: Samuel Sneed   **Patient Weight:** 40 kg
Patient ID#: 234906

Amino Acid: 2.5%
Dextrose: 25%

Additives:
NaCl 6 mEq/L   Ca Gluconate 20 mEq/L
Na Acetate 24 mEq/L   Mg Sulfate 4.16 mEq/L
KCL 6 mEq/L   PTE-5 2mls
K Phosphate 14 mEq/L   MVI 5 mLs

TPN Infusion Rate: 80mLs/hr over 24 hours

Intravenous Fats 20%: 17 mLs/hr over 24 hours

Date/Time: 4/29/1400   **Physician:** Jeff Hughes

MEDICAL PROFILE

Patient: Samuel Sneed   **Patient Weight:** 40 kg   **Age:** 7 y/o

Present Illness: MVA, Post OP   **Allergies:** Penicillin (rash)

Medical History: Multiple episodes of otitis media

Labs: Na 133, K 3.7, Cl 97, C02 21, Cr 0.6, BUN 10, Glu 250, Mg 1.9, ICA 1.2, WBC 4400, H/H 12/36.1, Plat 275,000, Segs 65%, Bands 4%, CRP 1.1, Alk Phos 54, AST 10, ALT 15, T Bili 0.6, D Bili 0.1, I Bili 0.5, Total Prot 6.9, Alb 3.5

Medication Profile:

Date	Medication
4/27/1700	Ranitidine 40 mg iv q 8 h
4/27/1700	Cefazolin 2 gm iv q 6 h
4/27/1700	Morphine sulfate 2 mg iv q 2–4 h prn
4/27/1700	Ondansetron 0.3 mg iv q 8 h prn

16a. Administering which of Samuel's medications would most likely result in the appearance of a rash?

A. Morphine
B. Cefazolin
C. Ondansetron
D. Ranitidine

16b. Which of Samuel's medications should be added to his TPN?

A. Morphine
B. Cefazolin
C. Ondansetron
D. Ranitidine

16c. Cefazolin is most likely prescribed to Samuel for _____.

A. prophylaxis for infections that might result from TPN administration
B. treatment of suspected sepsis based on WBC and CRP values
C. prevention or treatment of potential post-op infections
D. treatment of recurring otitis media

16d. Samuel's cefazolin regimen should be modified to _____.

A. 500 mg iv q 8 h
B. 500 mg iv q 6 h
C. 1000 mg iv q 8 h
D. 1000 mg iv q 6 h

16e. Samuel is most likely prescribed ondansetron for _____.

A. post-op nausea and vomiting
B. cefazolin-induced gastrointestinal upset
C. treatment of MVI-associated nausea and vomiting
D. nausea and vomiting associated with high-dextrose TPN therapy

16f. A more appropriate dose of ondansetron for Samuel is _____.

A. 3 mg
B. 3 mcg
C. 6 mg
D. 6 mcg

16g. What is the basal daily fluid requirement for a 40 kg patient such as Samuel?

A. 400 mLs
B. 1000 mLs
C. 1500 mLs
D. 1900 mLs

16h. Which of the following statements is true regarding centrally administered total parenteral nutrition?

A. Most commonly infused via ulnar or carotid vein
B. Osmolarity of infused solution should not exceed 900 mOsm/L
C. Requires high volumes to provide adequate caloric requirements
D. May be used for long-term nutritional support

16i. How many milliliters of a 10% amino acid solution are needed to prepare Samuel's TPN?

A. 120 mL
B. 240 mL
C. 360 mL
D. 480 mL

16j. Which of the following sources are typically included in calculating the total caloric intake from total parenteral nutrition?

A. Carbohydrate, fat, and protein
B. Carbohydrate and fat
C. Carbohydrate and protein
D. Fat and protein

16k. Approximately how many calories are provided from the dextrose component of Samuel's TPN?

A. 1400
B. 1600
C. 1900
D. 2100

16l. The most common fungus cultured from intravenous fat emulsions is _____.

A. *Candida albicans*
B. *Aspergillosis*
C. *Histoplasmosis*
D. *Malassezia furfur*

16m. Which of the following is most likely to be prescribed to Samuel?

    A. Sucralfate
    B. Fluconazole
    C. Magnesium sulfate
    D. Insulin

16n. Which of the following additives should be adjusted in Samuel's TPN?

    A. KCL
    B. NaCl
    C. Ca Gluconate
    D. Mg Sulfate

16o. Which of the following TPN additives would most likely create a solubility concern with phosphorus?

    A. Magnesium
    B. Potassium
    C. Sodium
    D. Calcium

16p. For every 100 calories metabolized in 24 hours, the average pediatric patient requires _____ mEq of sodium per day.

    A. 1–2
    B. 2–3
    C. 2–4
    D. 3–6

16q. For every 100 calories metabolized in 24 hours, the average pediatric patient requires _____ mEq of potassium per day.

    A. 1–2
    B. 2–3
    C. 2–4
    D. 3–6

CASE 17

PHYSICIAN ORDER

Patient Weight: <u>70 kg</u>

Begin risperidone 1 mg bid

Date/Time: <u>10/19/0415</u>
Physician: <u>Peter Barnes</u>

Patient Name: <u>Lee Carlisle</u>
Patient ID #: <u>245278</u>

MEDICAL PROFILE

Patient: Lee Carlisle

Patient Weight: 70 kg   **Age:** 17 y/o

Present Illness: Psychotic episode

Allergies: None

Medical History: Schizophrenia

Labs: Na 138, K 3.8, Cl 111, C02 24, Cr 0.7, BUN 10, Glu 135, Mg 2.2, WBC 4000, H/H 12.5/37.3, Plat 349000, Segs 45%, Bands 0%, Lymphs 26%, Monos 7%, CRP 0.7, Alk Phos 89, AST 17, ALT 18, T Bili 0.4, D Bili 0.3, I Bili 0.1, Total Prot 6.2, Alb 4.1

Medication Profile:

Date	Medication
10/19/0400	Haloperidol 5 mg iv q 4 h prn
10/19/0400	Lorazepam iv q 4 h prn

17a. Which of the following statements is true regarding schizophrenia?

　A. The onset is most commonly in early adolescence or late adulthood
　B. The onset tends to occur earlier in females
　C. Increasing evidence suggests a genetic basis for schizophrenia
　D. The term schizophrenia is synonymous with "split personality"

17b. Which of the following is classified as a "positive" symptom associated with schizophrenia?

　A. Alogia
　B. Anhedonia
　C. Social withdrawal
　D. Delusions

17c. Which of the following agents would most likely relieve both positive and negative symptoms associated with schizophrenia?

　A. Haloperidol
　B. Olanzapine
　C. Chlorpromazine
　D. Thioridazine

17d. Antipsychotic agents affect which of the following receptors?

　A. Dopamine
　B. Serotonin
　C. Histamine
　D. A and B only
　E. A, B, and C

17e. Which of Lee's prescribed medications is classified as a traditional or typical antipsychotic?

A. Haloperidol
B. Risperidone
C. Lorazepam
D. A and B only
E. A, B, and C

17f. Compared with low-potency traditional antipsychotic agents, which of the following adverse effects tends to occur more commonly with the high-potency agents?

A. Sedation
B. EPS
C. Anticholinergic effects
D. Orthostasis

17g. Which of the following medications is most closely related to risperidone?

A. Thioridazine
B. Chlorpromazine
C. Fluphenazine
D. Olanzapine

17h. Extrapyramidal adverse effects are believed to result from the blockade of _____ receptors by antipsychotic agents.

A. dopamine
B. histamine
C. muscarinic
D. serotonin

17i. Administering which of the following antipsychotic agents would be least likely to result in extrapyramidal side effects?

A. Haloperidol
B. Risperidone
C. Olanzapine
D. Quetiapine

17j. Which of the following extrapyramidal side effects is the most concerning and occurs late in onset relative to the initiation of antipsychotic therapy?

A. Dystonias
B. Pseudoparkinsonism
C. Akathisia
D. Tardive dyskinesia

17k. Which of the following is an antimuscarinic agent that may be prescribed to treat extrapyramidal side effects?

A. Amantadine
B. Benztropine
C. Diphenhydramine
D. Clonazepam

17l. Which of the following is true regarding Lee's haloperidol therapy?

A. It should only be administered orally or intramuscularly
B. The lactate formulation should be dispensed by the pharmacy
C. The lorazepam should be discontinued before initiating haloperidol therapy
D. The dose should be changed to 5 mcg iv q 4 h prn

17m. Which of the following dosage forms of risperidone could be potentially dispensed to Lee?

A. Tablets
B. Oral solution
C. Injectable solution
D. A and B only
E. A, B, and C

17n. For Lee, a reasonable targeted risperidone dosage regimen on day 3 of therapy would be _____.

A. 1 mg tid
B. 2 mg bid
C. 3 mg bid
D. 4 mg bid

17o. Initially, the maximum single dose of lorazepam that should be prescribed to Lee is _____ milligrams.

A. 1
B. 2
C. 3
D. 4

CASE 18

PHYSICIAN ORDER

Patient Weight: <u>13 kg</u>

Albumin 5% 12.5 gms iv

Date/Time: <u>8/23/1400</u>
Physician: <u>Ben Thompson</u>

Patient Name: <u>Carrie Phipps</u>
Patient ID #: <u>897278</u>

MEDICAL PROFILE

Patient: Carrie Phipps

Patient Weight: 13 kg   **Age:** 4 y/o

Present Illness: Nephrotic syndrome

Allergies: Sulfur

Medical History: Unremarkable

Labs: Na 134, K 3.9, Cl 107, C02 22.1, Cr 1.1, BUN 36, Glu 75, Mg 2.6, ICA .99, WBC 10400, H/H 14.5/43.2, Plat 322,000, Segs 58%, Bands 1%, Lymphs 33%, Monos 10.4%, CRP 2.3, Alk Phos 74, Chol 220, Alb 1.9

UA: SG 1.020, pH 6, Glucose 100, Blood Large, Protein > 300, Bacteria 1+

Cultures: Pending

Medication Profile:

Date	Medication
8/23/1200	Ceftriaxone 650 mg iv qd
8/23/1200	Prednisone 5 mg po qid
8/23/1200	Furosemide 13 mg iv q 6 h
8/23/1200	Lansoprazole 30 mg po qd

18a. Which of the following is consistent with nephrotic syndrome?

 A. Proteinuria
 B. Hypoproteinemia
 C. Hypercholesterolemia
 D. A and B only
 E. A, B, and C

18b. Which of the following is a possible complication associated with nephrotic syndrome.

 A. Pulmonary edema
 B. Oliguria
 C. Scrotal edema
 D. A and B only
 E. A, B, and C

18c. Which of the following lab values is likely to be decreased in Carrie?

   A. Triglycerides
   B. Oncotic pressure
   C. Thrombin
   D. Serum potassium

18d. The primary reason for prescribing albumin to Carrie is to _____.

   A. provide nutrition until she is able to eat by mouth
   B. increase intravascular volume
   C. decrease intravascular volume
   D. decrease renal perfusion

18e. A drug commonly prescribed with albumin is _____.

   A. Lasix
   B. Aldactone
   C. Procardia
   D. Tenormin

18f. As prescribed, how many milliliters of albumin are required to provide Carrie with her dose?

   A. 50 mL
   B. 100 mL
   C. 125 mL
   D. 250 mL

18g. A more appropriate albumin regimen for Carrie would be albumin _____.

   A. 5%, 130 mL iv
   B. 5%, 25 gms iv
   C. 25%, 12.5 gms iv
   D. 25%, 25 gms iv

18h. In the event Carrie's allergy is confirmed, which of the following would be the best substitute for her Lasix therapy?

   A. Bumex
   B. Edecrin
   C. HydroDIURIL
   D. Maxzide

18i. Which of the following is true of the furosemide prescribed for Carrie?

   A. Primarily acts at the ascending loop of Henle to inhibit chloride reabsorption
   B. The dose should be adjusted to 1.3 mg
   C. Should be discontinued and replaced with a thiazide diuretic
   D. A and B only
   E. A, B, and C

18j. A more appropriate prednisone regimen for Carrie would be _____.

   A. 13 mg po qd
   B. 13 mg po bid
   C. 25 mg po qd
   D. 25 mg po bid

18k. Which of the following medications has served as an alternative treatment for steroid-resistant nephrotic syndrome?

   A. Cyclophosphamide
   B. Cyclosporine
   C. Mycophenolate mofetil
   D. A and B only
   E. A, B, and C

18l. Which of the following drugs is most closely related to lansoprazole?

   A. Protonix
   B. Reglan
   C. Zantac
   D. Carafate

18m. Carrie's lansoprazole dose should be adjusted to _____.

   A. 7.5 mg po bid
   B. 15 mg po qd
   C. 15 mg po bid
   D. 30 mg po bid

CASE 1

1a (B) Kawasaki Syndrome (KS) is an acute, febrile, multisystem vasculitis that affects young children. Eighty percent of patients are younger than 5 years and it rarely affects children older than 8 years. Incidence rates are highest for children of Japanese and Korean ancestry and it occurs more commonly in males than in females with a ratio of ~ 1.5:1.

1b. (E) Although the etiology of KS is unknown, several have been hypothesized. These include rug shampoos, Epstein-Barr virus, a toxin from *Propionibacterium* acnes, herpes viruses 6 and 7, human parvovirus, Yersinia, and toxic shock syndrome toxin-1-producing *staphylococci*.

1c. (B) Cardiac involvement is the most important manifestation of KS. Coronary vasculitis manifested by dilatation or aneurysm formation in coronary arteries occurs in 10–40% of untreated patients. Pericarditis, myocarditis, endocarditis, heart failure, and arrhythmias may also be present.

1d. (D) The classical diagnosis of KS includes a fever for 5 or more days and 4 of the following: Bilateral conjunctival injections, changes in the mucosa of the oropharynx (i.e., strawberry-colored tongue), changes in peripheral extremities (i.e., edema, rash), rash (primarily truncal), and cervical lymphadenopathy.

1e. (E) Laboratory values consistent with KS include elevated markers of inflammation (i.e., sedimentation rate, C-reactive protein), elevated white blood cell count, high platelet counts, mild-to-moderate anemia, hypoalbuminemia, and elevated bilirubin and liver enzymes.

1f. (E) The primary goals in the treatment of KS are to control the acute inflammatory process including reducing the inflammation in the myocardium and in the coronary arteries and preventing thrombosis by inhibiting platelet aggregation.

1g. (E) Other trade names for intravenous immune globulin (IVIG) include Gammagard, Gammar, Polygam, and Iveegam.

1h. (E) Possible adverse effects from IVIG include flushing, tachycardia, hypotension, chills, fever, headache, nausea, chest tightness, sweating, and hypersensitivity reactions.

1i. (B) The preferred dose of IVIG for KS is a single dose of 2 gm/kg. Therefore, for Tina, 2 gm/kg × 11 kg = 22 gms. A dose of 400 mg/kg iv qd × 4 days has also been used.

1j. (D) The 2 gm/kg dose of IVIG is typically infused over 12 hours.

1k. (E) The mechanism of action of aspirin involves inhibition of prostaglandin synthesis subsequently resulting in analgesia and decreased inflammation. It also acts on the hypothalamus heat-regulating center to reduce fever.

1l. (E) Adverse effects of aspirin are related to its inhibition of prostaglandins. Such effects include gastrointestinal discomfort, ulceration and bleeding, decreased kidney function, and bronchospasms.

1m. (D) During the acute phase of KS, there appears to be decreased bioavailability of aspirin given the excessive doses needed to attain therapeutic concentrations. There is also evidence of an increase in unbound aspirin concentrations that may explain why lower doses and corresponding concentrations of aspirin may also be therapeutic.

1n. (D) A serum concentration of aspirin between 20–25 mg/dL appears to provide adequate anti-inflammatory effects.

1o. (D) During the acute phase of KS, the typical aspirin dose is 80–100 mg/kg/day divided every 6 hours. Therefore, for Tina, four baby aspirin tablets (81 mg each) every 6 hours would provide her with 243 mg per dose or 972 mg/day or 88 mg/kg/day (972 mg/11 kg = 88 mg/kg).

1p. (A) After the acute phase of KS and in the absence of fever, the aspirin dose may be decreased to an antiplatelet dose of 3–5 mg/kg/day. Therefore, 40 mg (~ 1/2 of a baby aspirin) once a day would provide Tina with ~ 3.5 mg/kg/day (40 mg/11 kg = 3.6 mg/kg).

1q. (C) Reye Syndrome is a potentially fatal event that may occur if aspirin is administered to children in the presence of a viral process (i.e., chicken pox, influenza). Therefore, in this case, the aspirin should be discontinued during the viral episode and dipyridamole, an antiplatelet agent, may be substituted.

1r. (E) Depending on the extent of coronary involvement in KS patients, continued or chronic therapy with antiplatelet and anticoagulants may be warranted. Such agents might include aspirin, dipyridamole, warfarin, and/or heparin.

CASE 2

2a. (B) Although most pneumonias in the pediatric age group are caused by viruses, *Streptococcus pneumoniae* is a major cause of bacterial pneumonias.

2b. (B) Recently, increased antibiotic resistance has been demonstrated with *Streptococcus pneumoniae* with the mechanism involving changes in penicillin-binding sites of the transpeptidases. Such resistance may be overcome by the use of higher doses of penicillins.

2c. (B) *Streptococcus pneumoniae* develops resistance to the macrolides via alteration of the 50S ribosome or by the presence of efflux pumps.

2d. (D) The respective trade and generic names are Claforan (cefotaxime), Fortaz (ceftazidime), Mefoxin (cefoxitin), and Rocephin (ceftriaxone).

2e. (C)

2f. (C) The mechanism of action of all the cephalosporins (i.e., Rocephin) involves the inhibition of bacterial cell-wall synthesis.

2g. (D) Rocephin is usually active against a number of gram-positive and gram-negative bacteria, but not against atypicals such as *Mycoplasma*.

2h. (C) The typical non-meningitic pediatric dose of Rocephin is 50 mg/kg iv qd. Therefore, John should receive 50 mg/kg × 25 kg = 1250 mg iv qd.

2i. (C) For the treatment of severe infections such as meningitis, the maximum recommended pediatric dose of Rocephin is 50 mg/kg iv q 12 hours with a maximum of 4 grams per day. Therefore, this would calculate to 5000 mg for a 50-kg child (50 mg/kg × 50 kg = 2500 mg q 12 h = 5000 mg per day). However, in this case, the child would receive 2000 mg iv q 12 hours, the maximum recommended amount per dose and per day.

2j. (C) Although vancomycin is mostly prescribed for *Staphylococcal* infections, it may be used for additional coverage against potentially resistant *Streptococcus*.

2k. (B) A half-life is defined as the time required for a drug concentration to decrease by one-half. John's vancomycin concentration decreased from 18 mcg/mL to 4.5 mcg/mL in 6 hours. Therefore, it decreased by 1/2 twice (18-9-4.5) during this time representing 2 half-lives in a 6-hour period or one half-life equaling 3 hours.

2l. (C) Most agree that vancomycin troughs between 5–10 mg/L or mcg/mL are adequate, although troughs between 5–15 mg/L have also been recommended.

2m. (B) In the presence of "normal" renal function, a reasonable initial pediatric dosing regimen of vancomycin would be 20 mg/kg iv q 8 hours. For John, 20 mg/kg × 25 kg = 500 mg iv q 8 hours.

2n. (B) Red Man Syndrome is a histamine-mediated reaction to vancomycin that manifests as a rash on the upper body (face, neck, trunk, and arms), pruritus, tachycardia, and hypotension that is often due to a rapid infusion rate. Slowing the infusion rate and/or administering an antihistamine is often helpful in the prevention of subsequent occurrences.

2o. (A) The respective trade and generic names are Zithromax (azithromycin), Biaxin (clarithromycin), E-mycin (erythromycin), and Zyban (bupropion).

2p. (C) Although technically an azalide, azithromycin is typically categorized as a macrolide antibiotic.

2q. (C)

2r. (B) Other drugs classified as macrolides include clarithromycin and erythromycin.

2s. (D) Although azithromycin has activity against certain gram-positive and gram-negative bacteria, it is a preferred drug for the treatment of *Mycoplasma*.

2t. (B) The pediatric intravenous dose of azithromycin is typically 10 mg/kg iv qd. Therefore, for John, 10 mg/kg × 25 kg = 250 mg iv qd.

CASE 3

3a. (E) Factors or conditions that predispose patients to aspiration pneumonia include decreased levels of consciousness, dysphagia, neurologic diseases, alcoholism, cerebrovascular accidents, esophageal disorders, nasogastric tube feeding, and general anesthesia.

3b. (E) The normal oral flora consists primarily of anaerobes (Bacteroides, Fusobacterium, *Peptostreptococcus*) and aerobes (*Streptococci*).

3c. (E) The oropharynx of hospitalized patients is often

colonized with gram-negative bacilli including *Klebsiella*, *Enterobacter*, and *Pseudomonas*. *Staphylococcus aureus*, a gram-positive bacteria, may also be present.

3d. (B) Expectorated sputum contains large numbers of indigenous anaerobes and positive blood cultures are uncommon in conjunction with anaerobic pneumonia. Therefore, tracheal aspiration or a bronchial brush provides more reliable results for a possible aspiration pneumonia.

3e. (D) Azithromycin was most likely prescribed for its activity against *Mycoplasma*. A negative IgM result for *Mycoplasma* indicates the absence of an acute infection, and therefore, it would be prudent to discontinue the azithromycin.

3f. (D) The respective generic and brand names are cefotaxime (Claforan), ceftazidime (Fortaz), cefixime (Suprax), and cefotaxime (Claforan).

3g. (C)

3h. (D) Cefotaxime lacks activity against *Mycoplasma* and most anaerobes, and provides no additional benefit to Timentin's coverage.

3i. (E) Timentin has excellent activity against many gram-positive and gram-negative bacteria as well as anaerobes. Therefore, it is widely used in the treatment of aspiration pneumonia.

3j. (D) A reasonable dose of Timentin for Bobby would be 200–300 mg/kg/day divided every 6 hours. Therefore, 1250 mg iv q 6 h would be appropriate (1250 mg × 4 = 5000mg/day; 5000 mg/17 kg = 294 mg/kg/day).

3k. (B) The most concerning toxic effect from an overdose of penicillins or cephalosporins is neurological, often manifested as seizure activity.

3l. (B) Timentin contains a high content of sodium, ~ 4.75 mEq/gram.

3m. (B) The adult dose and maximum recommended single dose of Timentin is 3.1 grams (Ticarcillin 3 grams, Clavulanic acid 0.1 gram).

3n. (A) Like Timentin, Zosyn (piperacillin/tazobactam) is an extended spectrum penicillin that provides similar antibacterial coverage.

3o. (D) Diarrhea is a common adverse effect from ampicillin therapy and does not indicate the presence of an allergy. Such documentation should be removed from Bobby's medical record.

CASE 4

4a. (D) The basic defect associated with cystic fibrosis (CF) is a mutation in the gene responsible for the chloride conductance channel referred to as the CF transmembrane conductance regulator (CFTR). The gene is located on the long arm of chromosome 7. Although many mutations are present at this locus, the most common mutation, delta F-508, accounts for 70% of the mutant CF alleles.

4b. (E) The classic triad associated with CF is elevated sweat chloride concentrations, pancreatic dysfunction, and pulmonary disease.

4c. (E) During infancy, meconium ileus, meconium peritonitis, prolonged jaundice, and failure to thrive should prompt investigation into the possibility of a patient with CF.

4d. (E) The sweat test is performed by iontophoresis of pilocarpine into the skin to stimulate sweating with a chloride concentration of greater than 60 mEq/L indicative of CF. Chronic pulmonary infections and pancreatic dysfunction, resulting in malabsorption of fats, are also evident in CF patients.

4e. (C) The lungs of CF patients usually harbor *Staphylococcus aureus* and *Haemophilus influenzae* initially with *Pseudomonas aeruginosa* becoming a common pathogen as the disease progresses.

4f. (C) Nebcin, the trade name of the antibiotic tobramycin, is an aminoglycoside prescribed mostly for the treatment of gram-negative bacteria such as *Pseudomonas*.

4g. (D) To achieve adequate concentrations and therapeutic benefit, cystic fibrosis (CF) patients require higher doses of antibiotics than do non-CF patients. Normal pediatric dosing of tobramycin is 7.5 mg/kg/day whereas CF patients often require 9–10 mg/kg/day.

4h. (B) Half-life = 0.693/Ke, where Ke (elimination rate constant) = ln C1/C2 divided by Δ t where C1 and C2 are concentrations and Δ t is the time between the two concentrations. For Heath, ln 5/0.5 divided by 6.5 hours (0500 to 1130) = 0.354; 0.693/0.354 = 1.9 hours.

4i. (D) Since tobramycin exhibits first-order kinetics, a ratio may be used with his existing tobramycin concentrations to calculate a dose to achieve a desired concentration provided the dosing interval remains constant. Hence, 120 mg/x = 5 mcg/mL/7.5 mcg/mL; x = 180 mg.

4j. (B) Oxacillin is a penicillin antibiotic with excellent coverage against *Staphylococcus aureus*; however, it is not active against methicillin resistant *Staphylococcus aureus* (MRSA). In the absence of MRSA in Heath, oxacillin would be a excellent substitute for vancomycin.

4k. (E)

4l. (B) Pulmozyme is a deoxyribonuclease enzyme produced by recombinant gene technology that improves mucociliary clearance by hydrolyzing extracellular deoxyribonucleic acid (DNA) present in airway secretions.

4m. (C) The correct dose of Pulmozyme is 2.5 mg via nebulization once daily. Although Pulmozyme may be dosed twice daily, studies indicate once daily dosing is as effective for most patients.

4n. (B) ADEK contains the fat soluble vitamins A, D, E, and K that may be deficient in CF patients. It also contains thiamine, ascorbic acid, folic acid, riboflavin, niacin, pyridoxine, cyanocobalamin, biotin, pantothenic acid, zinc, and beta carotene. Children older than 10 years receive two tablets daily. The tablets must be crushed or chewed thoroughly.

4o. (C) The pancreatic enzyme preparations (i.e., Pancrease) contain the enzymes lipase, amylase, and protease. Dosing is based on the lipase concentration with the dose calculated per grams of ingested fat or per patient weight in kilograms. In general, patients require 500–4000 lipase units per gram of fat or an initial dose of 1000 lipase units per kilogram of body weight per meal.

4p. (D) Pancrease MT 16 contains 16,000 units of lipase per capsule.

4q. (E) Pancrease is usually well tolerated; however, it may cause constipation, mucosal irritation, intussusception, or rarely, proximal colonic strictures.

CASE 5

5a. (D) Acetaminophen dose = 225 mg. Stock solution = 160 mg/5 mL; 160 mg/5 mL = 225 mg/x; x = 7.03 mLs.

5b. (B) Acetaminophen with codeine elixir contains codeine 12 mg/5 mL. Therefore, 12 mg/5 mL = x/3 mL; x = 7.2 mg.

5c. (B) Acetaminophen with codeine elixir contains acetaminophen 120 mg/5 mL. Therefore, 120 mg/5 mL = x/3 mLs; x = 72 mg.

5d. (C) Both imipenem/cilastatin and meropenem are classified as carbapenems.

5e. (A) The respective generic and trade names are imipenen/cilastatin (Primaxin), lisinopril (Prinvil), pentamidine (Pentam), and ampicillin (Principen).

5f. (E) The carbapenems are broad spectrum antibiotics that are active against most gram-negative, gram-positive, and anaerobic bacteria.

5g. (B) Imipenem is hydrolyzed and inactivated by dehydropeptidase, a renal brush-border enzyme. Cilastatin, a dehydropeptidase inhibitor, prevents this renal metabolism of imipenem.

5h. (B) The pediatric dose of imipenem/cilastatin is 60–100 mg/kg/day with a maximum of 4 grams per day.

5i. (D) Risk factors for the development of seizures while receiving imipenem/cilastatin include a history of seizures, central nervous system lesions, renal insufficiency, and excessive doses. For Daryl, meropenem (Merrem), also a carbapenem, would be a better choice.

5j. (B) The respective generic and trade names are trandolapril (Mavik), meropenem (Merrem), cefepime (Maxipime), and meprobamate (Miltown).

5k. (A) Meropenem is indicated for the treatment of meningitis in a dose of 40 mg/kg every 8 hours with a maximum recommended dose of 2 grams every 8 hours. It is renally eliminated, and therefore dosage adjustments are needed in the presence of renal insufficiency.

5l. (D) Meropenem and imipenem/cilastatin share similar antibacterial activity with meropenem being more active against gram-negative bacteria. Neither are active against methicillin resistant *Staphylococcus aureus*, MRSA.

5m. (C) The correct dose of meropenem for Daryl is 20 mg/kg iv every 8 hours. Therefore, the dose should be 20 mg/kg × 15 kg = 300 mg iv q 8 h.

5n. (C)

5o. (B) Serum sickness appears to occur more often with Ceclor than with other β-lactam antibiotics. It is characterized by fever, lymphadenopathy, arthralgias, cutaneous eruptions, gastrointestinal disturbances, proteinuria, and malaise.

CASE 6

6a. (D) Epogen, erythropoietin, is a colony-stimulating factor that induces erythropoiesis by stimulating the division and differentiation of committed erythroid cells. Adequate iron stores are needed to optimize the response to Epogen therapy.

6b. (A) Iron sulfate consists of 20% elemental iron. Therefore, a dose of 125 mg 3 times a day of iron sulfate = 375 mg/day or 75 mg of elemental iron (375 mg × 0.2 = 75 mg).

6c. (E) The major adverse effects of oral iron therapy involve the gastrointestinal system (dark stools, constipation, irritation, etc.).

6d. (B) Approximately 90% of erythropoietin is produced in the kidney and the remainder is produced in the liver.

6e. (D) Epogen is administered either by subcutaneous or intravenous injection.

6f. (A) In an attempt to optimize Epogen therapy, the patient should have a serum ferritin concentration >100 ng/dL and a transferrin saturation > 20%.

6g. (D) A hematocrit of 32 to 38% is often targeted during Epogen therapy. Therefore, considerations to discontinue therapy might be addressed when hematocrit concentrations approach the upper values.

6h. (E) Iron deficiency is often associated with an inadequate response to Epogen therapy. Infection and inflammation may block the release of iron from the reticuloendothelial cells resulting in decreased effectiveness of Epogen.

6i. (E) Epogen is usually well tolerated; adverse effects are mainly limited to flu-like symptoms. Other side effects that may occur as a result of increasing red cell mass include iron deficiency, hypertension, and seizures.

6j. (C) Although a range of doses have been used in pediatric patients, most have received between 100–400 units/kg 3 times a week. Therefore, Susan might receive 2500 units (2500 units/18 kg = 139 units/kg) three times a week.

6k. (D) PhosLo is a product that contains calcium acetate. As a result of Susan's elevated phosphate concentration, it might be desirable to prescribe a phosphate binder such as PhosLo to lower her phosphate concentration.

6l. (A) Fortaz is primarily eliminated via the kidneys and therefore requires a dosage adjustment in the presence of renal insufficiency. For Susan, it would most likely be dosed every 1 to 2 days.

6m. (C) *Staphylococcus epidermidis* is a common nosocomial pathogen that is often highly resistant to antibiotics commonly prescribed for gram-positive bacteria with the exception of vancomycin. For mixed infections, ceftazidime is often prescribed with vancomycin. Oxacillin is metabolized via the liver and often does not necessitate dosage adjustments in the presence of renal dysfunction.

6n. (A) Vancomycin is eliminated via the kidneys and requires close monitoring of drug concentrations in the presence of renal insufficiency. However, regardless of the degree of renal dysfunction, the initial dose of vancomycin remains unchanged from that of a patient with normal renal function. Therefore, her first dose should be 360 mg (20 mg/kg × 18 kg = 360 mg) as prescribed.

6o. (C) The best strategy for dosing vancomycin in the presence of renal insufficiency is to administer one dose after which a couple of concentrations are obtained to perform a pharmacokinetic analysis to guide future dosing.

CASE 7

7a. (C) Procardia XL is an extended-release preparation and therefore should not be crushed or chewed. It is classified as a calcium-channel antagonist. Adalat CC is another brand name of the same active ingredient, nifedipine.

7b. (D) Luis is prescribed calcitriol for the management of hypocalcemia common to patients receiving dialysis. It promotes the intestinal absorption and the renal retention of calcium.

7c. (E) Calcitriol, 1,25 dihydroxycholecalciferol, is the active form of vitamin D. Brand names include Rocaltrol and Calcijex.

7d. (C) Enalapril is a prodrug that is converted in-vivo to enalaprilat, the injectable form of enalapril. Capoten (captopril) is also an angiotensin-converting enzyme inhibitor, but is not available parenterally.

7e. (E) Potential adverse effects from enalapril, as well as the other angiotensin-converting enzyme inhibitors, include hypotension, hyperkalemia, cough, and rarely, angioedema.

7f. (D)

7g. (B)

7h. (A) The most common adverse effects from oral clonidine include drowsiness, bradycardia, dry mouth, dizziness, and rebound hypertension.

7i. (A) Catapres TTS-1 is a transdermal patch of clonidine that provides 0.1 mg of clonidine over 24 hours. The patch is replaced every 7 days. The patches are also available as TTS –2 and TTS-3 systems.

7j. (C) Luis is prescribed 0.1 mg of clonidine daily. Therefore, 0.1 mg = 100 mcg (1 mg = 1000 mcg); 100 mcg/20 kg = 5 mcg/kg/day.

7k. (B) Calcium carbonate contains the most elemental calcium per gram relative to the other calcium salts available. Amount of elemental calcium (mg) per 1 gram of salt: Calcium carbonate – 400, Calcium chloride – 270, Calcium lactate – 130, Calcium gluconate – 90.

7l. (D) Luis has an elevated phosphate concentration secondary to his chronic renal disease, and therefore, it may be desirable to prescribe a phosphate binder of which calcium-containing products are often used. Calcium acetate (PhosLo) is a more effective phosphate binder than either calcium carbonate or calcium citrate and might be of more benefit in lowering Luis' phosphate.

7m. (C) Calcium carbonate contains 40% elemental calcium. Therefore, 500 mg tid = 1500 mg/day; 1500 mg × 0.4 (40%) = 600 mg elemental calcium; 600 mg/20 kg = 30 mg/kg/day of elemental calcium.

7n. (B) Shohl's solution is an alkalizing agent used for the treatment of chronic metabolic acidosis.

7o. (A) Shohl's solution contains sodium citrate and citric acid.

7p. (B) Citrate is metabolized to bicarbonate by the liver so that each mL of Shohl's solution provides 1 mEq of bicarbonate. Therefore, Luis is receiving 45 mLs (15 mL tid) of Shohl's solution per day that is equivalent to 45 mEq's of bicarbonate; 45 mEq bicarbonate/20 kg = 2.3 mEq/kg or ~ 2.

7q. (D) Both nifedipine and nicardipine are dihydropyridine-calcium antagonists. Both diltiazem and verapamil are non-dihydropyridine calcium antagonists.

7r. (A) Nifedipine is an antihypertensive agent that acts rapidly when administered sublingually. However, nifedipine exhibits negligible sublingual absorption with its effects predominately resulting from swallowing the appropriate measured aliquot that is obtained from the fluid-filled capsules.

7s. (A) Common side effects from nifedipine therapy include hypotension, flushing, reflex tachycardia, and edema.

7t. (C) The dosing range of nifedipine most commonly used in pediatric patients is 0.25 to 0.5 mg/kg/dose. Side effects appear to occur less with the use of lower doses without compromising efficacy. Therefore, an initial dose of 0.25 mg/kg would be reasonable for Luis. Hence, 0.25 mg/kg × 20 kg = 5 mg.

CASE 8

8a. (E) An infant or young child almost always has a secondary cause for hypertension. Such causes include renal and cardiovascular disease, seizures, volume overload, anxiety, trauma, and medications. Essential hypertension is most common during adolescence.

8b. (A) Furosemide is a loop diuretic that acts on the ascending limb of the loop of Henle to block the Na-K-2Cl cotransporter. Other loops include bumetanide, torsemide, and ethacrynic acid.

8c. (E) Other potential side effects of furosemide include hypomagnesemia, hyperglycemia, increased triglycerides and cholesterol, and ototoxicity.

8d. (A) Both bumetanide (Bumex) and furosemide (Lasix) are loop diuretics.

8e. (C) Furosemide is ~ 50% bioavailable. Therefore, the oral dose must be approximately double the intravenous dose to achieve the same effect. Since Jerry is prescribed furosemide 20 mg orally, an equivalent intravenous dose would be 10 mg, one-half the oral dose.

8f. (D) Chlorothiazide is a thiazide diuretic and unlike the loop diuretics, it results in retention of calcium by the kidney. Given Jerry's history of renal stones, it might be prudent to avoid loop diuretics that might lead to increased excretion of calcium stones.

8g. (A) Metolazone is a thiazide-like diuretic that acts to prevent sodium transport in the distal tubule by blocking the Na-Cl cotransporter. Hydrochlorothiazide is a thiazide diuretic with an identical mechanism of action.

8h. (B) Often diuretics with different sites of action are combined to increase diuresis. Metolazone, which primarily acts on the distal tubule, is often prescribed with furosemide, a loop diuretic, to enhance diuresis.

8i. (E) Spironolactone, amiloride, and triamterene are potassium-sparing diuretics that block sodium reabsorption in the collecting duct while preventing the loss of potassium. Therefore, potassium supplementation is cautioned in the presence of these diuretics.

8j. (A) Oral potassium chloride is a much safer mode of drug delivery compared with intravenous potassium. Intravenous potassium administration is associated with phlebitis and requires ECG monitoring. Side effects of oral potassium predominately involve the gastrointestinal system and include nausea, vomiting, abdominal pain, and ulcers. Oral potassium should be diluted in water or juice before administration.

8k. (B)

8l. (D) Side effects of β-adrenergic antagonists (i.e., propranolol) include bradycardia, syncope, CNS depression, bronchoconstriction, decreased exercise capacity, and decreased sexual potency.

8m. (E)

8n. (A) Unlike propranolol, atenolol is a β-1 selective adrenergic antagonist. Propranolol blocks both β-1 and β-2 receptors. With Jerry's history of asthma, it would be desirable to avoid the use of β-2 adrenergic blocking agents that could potentially exacerbate Jerry's asthma. Ideally, all β-adrenergic antagonists should be avoided in asthma patients.

8o. (B) Labetalol is a non-selective β-adrenergic antagonist and a selective α-1 adrenergic antagonist. It is available in both oral and intravenous dosage forms and is indicated for the treatment of hypertension.

CASE 9

9a. (D) Appendicitis is one of the most common conditions requiring emergency surgery in children. It occurs more commonly in males with the peak incidence being around 12 years of age. It is particularly difficult to diagnose in females because similar symptoms are associated with pelvic inflammatory disease, ovarian cysts, and ectopic pregnancy. Sudden relief of pain usually indicates perforation as the intraluminal pressure in the appendix is relieved.

9b. (B) Gentamicin is predominantly active against gram-negative aerobic bacteria.

9c. (A) Gentamicin exhibits concentration-dependent killing activity indicating that for optimal activity, peak concentrations well above the minimum inhibitory concentration are required.

9d. (A) Linda is receiving once daily dosing of gentamicin. The rationale for such dosing is to achieve high peak concentrations for optimal bactericidal effects and very low or often undetectable trough concentrations to reduce toxicity. The concentration obtained represents a peak concentration on the first dose and appears reasonable given that a dose of 7.5 mg/kg (225mg/30 kg = 7.5 mg/kg) was given. The volume of distribution for gentamicin in pediatric patients is ~ 0.25–0.3 L/kg. Therefore, using the equation: Concentration = Dose/Volume of Distribution, we have; Conc = 7.5 mg/kg/0.3 L/kg = 25 mg/L. A second concentration should be obtained before her second dose to ensure adequate elimination.

9e. (C) Once daily dosing of gentamicin should result in trough concentrations (concentration just prior to a dose) that are very low or undetectable.

9f. (B) The postantibiotic effect is the mechanism by which gentamicin's bactericidal activity continues in the presence of undetectable serum concentrations.

9g. (D) Nephrotoxicity and ototoxicity are the most concerning adverse effects of gentamicin therapy and are believed to be associated with drug accumulation in the respective organs. Therefore, once daily dosing, which often results in undetectable trough concentrations, is believed to reduce the incidence of such adverse effects.

9h. (C) Traditionally, gentamicin is initially prescribed as 2.5 mg/kg iv q 8 hours. Therefore, Linda would receive 2.5 mg/kg × 30 kg = 75 mg iv q 8 h.

9i. (B) Gentamicin is classified as an aminoglycoside as is tobramycin.

9j. (B) Acetaminophen with codeine contains 12 mg of codeine per 5 mLs. Linda is prescribed 1 teaspoonful which is equivalent to ~ 5 milliliters. Therefore, she will receive 12 mg per dose.

9k. (B)

9l. (C) The respective generic and trade names are cloxacillin (Cloxapen), clarithromycin (Biaxin), clindamycin (Cleocin), and cefotaxime (Claforan).

9m. (C) Clindamycin is active against gram-positive and anaerobic bacteria. In the case of appendicitis, it is prescribed mostly for its anaerobic activity.

9n. (B) Clindamycin is well known to result in overgrowth of Clostridium difficile and resultant pseudomembranous colitis.

9o. (E)

9p. (A) Both clindamycin and lincomycin are lincosamides.

9q. (A) Clindamycin is compatible with gentamicin and is often combined in the same intravenous solution, especially when both are dosed on an 8-hourly schedule.

9r. (B) Clindamycin dose = 400 mg and is available as a 150 mg/mL solution. Therefore, 150 mg/1 mL = 400 mg/x; x = 2.7 mL.

9s. (A) Clindamycin is typically dosed at 20–40 mg/kg/day divided every 6–8 hours; usually every 8 hours. Therefore, for Linda 400 mg iv q 8 h = 400 mg/30 kg = 13 mg/kg every 8 hours or 40 mg/kg/day.

9t. (C) Linda was most likely prescribed morphine in the event she needs additional pain relief not provided from the acetaminophen with codeine. Codeine is available parenterally and morphine would likely result in increased itching as it often results in histamine release.

CASE 10

10a. (C) The respective generic and trade names are famotidine (Pepcid), nizatidine (Axid), sucralfate (Carafate), and ranitidine (Zantac).

10b. (D) Sucralfate is an aluminum salt of sulfated sucrose that in the presence of gastric acid forms a complex that adheres to and protects damaged mucosa.

10c. (B) Sucralfate is an aluminum salt and because of potential accumulation, should be used cautiously in the presence of renal dysfunction.

10d. (B) Sucralfate is only available for oral administration and is most commonly dosed at 40–80 mg/kg/day divided every 6 hours. Therefore, 500 mg po q 6 hours = 2000 mg/day or 67 mg/kg/day (2000 mg/30 kg = 66.67 mg/kg).

10e. (A) The respective generic and trade names are metronidazole (Flagyl), ofloxacin (Floxin), bupropion (Zyban), and olanzapine (Zyprexa).

10f. (C) Metronidazole is a nitroimidazole antimicrobial indicated for anaerobic and protozoal infections.

10g. (A) Metronidazole is also prescribed as a component of multidrug regimens for *Helicobacter pylori*.

10h. (A) Peripheral neuropathy is a rare, but potentially serious adverse effect of long-term, moderate-to-high dose, metronidazole therapy. The neuropathy may persist for many months after drug discontinuation.

10i. (B) When metronidazole is combined with alcohol, a disulfiram-type reaction may occur resulting in nausea with possible severe vomiting.

10j. (B) Neutralized solutions of metronidazole are available in ready-to-use 5 mg/mL (500 mg) foil-covered containers to protect them from light. They should be stored at room temperature because refrigeration may result in precipitation.

10k. (B) During metronidazole therapy, white blood cell counts with differential should be obtained as neutropenia and leukopenia may occur.

10l. (A) Intravenous metronidazole is usually dosed at 30 mg/kg/day divided every 6 hours. Therefore, for Lisa, 30 mg/kg/day × 30 kg = 900 mg/day or 225 mg iv q 6 h (900 mg/4 doses = 225 mg/dose). A dosage of 250 mg iv q 6 h (1000 mg/day divided by 30 kg = 33 mg/kg/day) would also be reasonable as the 500 mg commercially available bag could be easily divided into two doses for Lisa without the need to discard excess drug.

10m. (A) Ampicillin is the drug of choice for *Listeria monocytogenes*. It is also active against select gram-positive, gram-negative, and anaerobic bacteria.

10n. (C) Reconstituted ampicillin solutions should be used within 1 hour. Normal saline is the preferred diluent for the reconstituted solutions as the resultant preparation is stable for ~ 8 hours versus 2 hours if a dextrose solution is used. Injectable ampicillin may be administered intramuscularly as well as intravenously.

10o. (B) For nonmeningitis, ampicillin is dosed at 100–200 mg/kg/day divided every 6 hours. There-fore, for Lisa, 1000 mg iv q 6 hours = 4000 mg/day or 133 mg/kg/day (4000 mg/30 kg = 133 mg/kg).

CASE 11

11a. (A) Tuberculosis is caused by the bacillus *Mycobacterium tuberculosis*. Most strains are slow growing with doubling times approaching 24 hours. Primary infection occurs from inhaling organisms contained in droplet nuclei.

11b. (C) The Ziehl-Neelsen or the fluorochrome stains are used for *M. tuberculosis*. After staining with carbol-fuchsin, mycobacteria retain a red color, despite alcohol washes, and are therefore referred to as acid fast bacilli or AFB.

11c. (B) The preferred skin test for tuberculosis is the Mantoux test that is performed by placing 5 tuberculin units of purified protein derivative (PPD) intracutaneously on the volar aspect of the forearm.

11d. (E) The PPD test should be read in 48–72 hours. For immunocompetent persons, an induration > 10 mm is considered positive; for HIV-infected patients and recent contacts of tuberculosis patients, > 5 mm is considered positive. Two products are available, Aplisol and Tubersol, with Tubersol being preferred due to more predictable results.

11e. (B) For latent tuberculosis, INH is usually prescribed for 6–9 months.

11f. (B) The addition of pyrazinamide (PZA) to INH and rifampin shortens the duration of therapy from 9 to 6 months.

11g. (E) The most common adverse effects from pyrazinamide therapy include GI distress, arthralgias, and elevated serum uric acid concentrations. Hepatotoxicity is the major limiting adverse effect, but occurs less often.

11h. (C) Rifampin is an inducer of the cytochrome P-450 isoenzyme system, and therefore, may increase the metabolism of theophylline necessitating the need for an increased dose of theophylline to maintain therapeutic concentrations.

11i. (D)

11j. (C) INH appears to exert its neurotoxic effects through enhanced elimination of pyridoxine, vitamin B6. Therefore, patients treated with INH may be prescribed supplemental pyridoxine.

11k. (D) The primary neurotoxic manifestation from INH therapy is peripheral neuropathy.

11l. (B) INH is dosed at 10–20 mg/kg/day in one or two doses. Therefore, 300 mg po qd would be appropriate for Robert (300 mg/20 kg = 15 mg/kg).

11m. (E) Rifampin is also active against *M. bovis* and *M. kansasii*. It also has activity against other nontuber-culous mycobacteria including *M. avium* complex.

11n. (C) Rifampin may be administered orally or parenterally. It is a potent inducer of the cytochrome P-450 isoenzyme system. Rifampin administration also results in urine, tears, and other bodily secretions exhibiting a red-orange color.

11o. (B) Ethambutol's major toxicity is retrobulbar neuritis and occurs more commonly with doses exceeding 30 mg/kg/day. Patients usually complain of a change in visual acuity and/or the inability to see the color green.

CASE 12

12a. (D) Arabinosylcytosine is also synonymous with Ara-C. Brand names include Cytosar-U and Tarabine PFS. CytoGam is the trade name for cytomegalovirus immune globulin.

12b. (A) Ara-C is converted intracellularly to an active metabolite, cytarabine triphosphate. Its mode of action involves inhibition of DNA polymerase resulting in inhibition of DNA synthesis. Ara-C has limited permeability across the blood-brain barrier. It may be administered intravenously, intramuscularly, subcutaneously, or intrathecally.

12c. (E) Major potential adverse effects associated with Ara-C include myelosuppression, nausea, vomiting, diarrhea, fever, hepatotoxicity, stomatitis, and alopecia.

12d. (D) Daunorubicin inhibits DNA and RNA synthesis by intercalating between DNA base pairs, uncoiling of the helix, and by steric obstruction.

12e. (C) Irreversible myocardial toxicity is the major concern with daunorubicin therapy and is more common as cumulative doses approach 550 mg/m^2 in adults or 300 mg/m^2 in pediatric patients.

12f. (D) Daunorubicin is metabolized to the active metabolite, daunorubicinol. A transient red-orange discoloration of the urine may occur up to 48 hours after a dose. The drug is irritating and should not be administered intramuscularly or subcutaneously.

12g. (A) Adriamycin is the trade name for doxorubicin, a drug similar to daunorubicin regarding mechanism of action and potential adverse effects.

12h. (D) Allopurinol inhibits xanthine oxidase thus preventing the conversion of hypoxanthine to xanthine and thus xanthine to uric acid.

12i. (A) Morphine sulfate may cause itching as a result of its ability to induce release of histamine. Benadryl, an antihistamine, may be used to treat this morphine-induced itching.

12j. (A) Vancomycin and ceftazidime are often used in combination to provide empiric broad antimicrobial coverage in neutropenic patients.

12k. (D) Studies have indicated that oncology patients often require higher than standard doses of vancomycin (i.e., 60–75 mg/kg/day) to achieve desired serum concentrations. Leonard is currently prescribed 60 mg/kg/day (3000 mg/day divided by 50 kg = 60 mg/kg/day), which is a reasonable dose pending concentrations.

12l. (E) Amphotericin-B administration can result in renal wasting of potassium and magnesium. Additionally, adequate sodium administration has been shown to decrease the incidence of amphotericin-B induced nephrotoxicity. Therefore, close monitoring of each of these is essential during amphotericin-B therapy.

12m. (B) "Lipid" formulations of amphotericin-B are most commonly prescribed for refractory fungal infections or when nephrotoxicity results from the use of amphotericin-B deoxycholate.

12n. (A)

12o. (C) Amphotericin-B's mechanism of action involves binding to sterols (ergosterol) in the fungal cell wall resulting in altered permeability, leakage of cell components, and thus, cell death.   ·

12p. (A) Meperidine administration has proven effective in reducing the rigors associated with amphotericin-B therapy.

12q. (D) The respective "amphotericin-B" products are as follows: Fungizone = amphotericin B deoxycholate, Amphotec = amphotericin B cholesteryl, Abelcet = amphotericin B lipid complex, Ambisone = liposomal amphotericin B.

12r. (C) Liposomal amphotericin B is typically dosed at 3–5 mg/kg as a single daily dose. Therefore, a dose of 200 mg (200 mg/50 kg = 4 mg/kg) iv qd would be appropriate for Leonard.

CASE 13

13a. (C) The prognosis from acute lymphoblastic leukemia (ALL) is less encouraging when diagnosis occurs in children younger than 1 year or older than 15 years of age. Fortunately, the leukemic cells of children with ALL are sensitive to chemotherapy. The platelet count of ALL patients varies from normal to extremely low with a mean of 50×10^9/L. Leukocyte counts typically range from 0.1 to 1600 $\times 10^9$/L.

13b. (D) Opiates, such as morphine, are associated with side effects including drowsiness, constipation, CNS depression, nausea/vomiting, miosis, vasodilation, tolerance, and dependence. When used appropriately for pain control, psychological dependence is not usually described.

13c. (A) Intravenous morphine sulfate is typically initially dosed at 0.05–0.1 mg/kg. The dose should be titrated based on response, adverse effects, and the development of tolerance. For Ben, a reasonable

initial dose would be 1.2 mg (0.05 mg/kg × 24 kg = 1.2 mg).

13d. (C) In the event a patient is prescribed analgesics on an "as needed" schedule and is being dosed consistently per the "as needed" dosing interval, it would be prudent to establish a scheduled dosing interval for the patient in an attempt to provide better pain relief. Too often, analgesics are prescribed at inappropriately low doses or are withheld because of concerns of adverse effects or the possibility of addiction. In this case, Ben's dose should be increased and a dosing interval established to allow him optimal analgesia.

13e. (A) On many hospital narcotic order forms, naloxone (a narcotic antagonist) is prescribed concurrently with an opiate so that it will be readily available in the event an overdose of the opiate occurs or the patient has an unexpected enhanced effect from the opiate.

13f. (B) Naloxone is usually dosed at 0.01 mg/kg with a maximum dose of 0.4 mg. For Ben, the dose would be 0.01 mg/kg × 24 kg = 0.24 mg.

13g. (C) Both Velban and Velsar are trade names for vinblastine, a drug similar to vincristine. Omnipen is a trade name for ampicillin.

13h. (C) Vincristine binds to the microtubular protein of the mitotic spindle resulting in cellular metaphase arrest.

13i. (E) The most common adverse effects of vincristine include alopecia, loss of deep tendon reflexes, and local ulceration if extravasation occurs. Others include jaw pain, peripheral neuropathy, and weakness. Although less common, inappropriate antidiuretic hormone secretion may occur.

13j. (C) For ALL, vincristine is typically dosed at 1–1.5 mg/m²/week for 3–6 weeks.

13k. (B)

13l. (A) Vincristine is a tissue irritant and should only be administered intravenously. Intrathecal administration has resulted in death.

13m. (A) The respective generic and trade names are asparaginase (Elspar), candesartan (Atacand), carboplatin (Paraplatin), and pegaspargase (Oncaspar).

13n. (D) Although anorexia, convulsions, and pancreatitis may result from asparaginase therapy, hypersensitivity reactions are more common. Therefore, an intradermal skin test should be performed before the initial dose and when therapy is reinitiated after an interval of 1 week or more.

13o. (B) For ALL, asparaginase is usually dosed at 6000–10,000 IU/m² IM three times a week. High dose therapy is 25,000 IU/m²/week IM for 9–20 weeks.

13p. (B) Compared with the intravenous route, the intramuscular administration of asparaginase is associated with less severe anaphylactoid reactions.

13q. (B) 10,000 units/2 mL = 5500 units/x; x = 1.1 mLs.

13r. (D) For ALL, prednisone is usually dosed at 40 mg/m²/day PO for 28 days (maximum dose = 60 mg). Alternatively, dexamethasone may be used at a dose of 6 mg/m²/day PO for 28 days.

13s. (E) Systemic corticosteroids, such as prednisone, have many potential adverse effects including adrenal suppression, gastric ulcers, Cushing's syndrome, immunosuppression, psychosis, cataracts, acne, osteoporosis, leukocytosis, hypertension, hyperglycemia, poor wound healing, growth retardation, and pancreatitis.

13t. (A) Intrathecal therapy with methotrexate is used in the treatment of ALL. For intrathecal administration, preservative-free methotrexate should be used.

CASE 14

14a. (D) The acronym "CHOP" is derived from the first letters of the drugs used: C: Cyclophosphamide; H: Hydroxydaunorubicin (Doxorubicin); O: Oncovin (Vincristine); P: Prednisone.

14b. (B) The respective generic and trade names are cytarabine (Cytosar), cyclophosphamide (Cytoxan), liothyronine (Cytomel), and ganciclovir (Cytovene).

14c. (B) Cyclophosphamide is an alkylating agent that acts to inhibit DNA synthesis.

14d. (E) Adverse effects associated with cyclophos-phamide include alopecia, myelosuppression, nausea, vomiting, metallic taste, hemorrhagic cystitis, and inappropriate ADH secretion.

14e. (A) To guard against hemorrhagic cystitis from cyclophosphamide therapy, aggressive hydration and adequate urination is recommended. It is recommended to be reconstituted with a preservative free diluent. The recommended final concentration of cyclophosphamide for administration is 20–25 mg/mL. It is available in

both an oral and intravenous dosage form.

14f. (B) In the urinary bladder, mesna acts to reduce the occurrence of hemorrhagic cystitis by binding to and detoxifying acrolein and other urotoxic metabolites of both ifosfamide and cyclophosphamide.

14g. (A) The respective generic and trade names are doxorubicin (Adriamycin), dexrazoxane (Zinecard), doxycycline (Doryx), and fluorouracil (Adrucil).

14h. (E) Adverse effects commonly associated with doxorubicin therapy include alopecia, myelosuppression, cardiac toxicity, nausea/vomiting, local ulceration, and a pink or red urine color.

14i. (D) Doxorubicin is a vesicant and therefore should only be administered intravenously.

14j. (D)

14k. (B) G-CSF is a 175-amino acid nonglycosylated protein derived from E-coli cultures that stimulates granulopoiesis and hence the production, maturation, and activation of neutrophils.

14l. (A) G-CSF is marketed as Neupogen (filgrastim). Prokine and Epogen are the trade name for GM-CSF and erythropoietin, respectively.

14m. (B) G-CSF may be given via the intravenous or subcutaneous route, but should not be administered 24 hours prior to or 24 hours following the administration of chemotherapy. An increase in the neutrophil count may be seen within 1–2 days of therapy. It is contraindicated in patients sensitive to *E. coli* derived products.

14n. (E) The most common adverse effects associated with G-CSF therapy are arthralgias, myalgias, medullary bone pain, headache, skin rash, fever, and itching. The bone pain can usually be managed with non-narcotic analgesics.

14o. (D) The usual dose of G-CSF is 5–10 mcg/kg once daily until the desired neutrophil count is achieved. Therefore, a reasonable starting dose for Heather would be 300 mcg sc qd (300 mcg/50 kg = 6 mcg/kg/day).

CASE 15

15a. (D) To assist in the diagnosis of pancreatitis, amylase and lipase concentrations should be obtained. Elevations of these enzymes are indicative of pancreatitis.

15b. (C) The belief that morphine induces spasms of the sphincter of Oddi to a greater degree than meperidine has been perpetuated over many years. Current evidence does not support this as both morphine and meperidine may restrict the flow at the sphincter of Oddi with an increase in bile pressure. No evidence exists supporting the use of meperidine in lieu of morphine for pain associated with pancreatitis.

15c. (C) The recommended initial intravenous dose of morphine sulfate is 0.05–0.1 mg/kg. Therefore, an initial 2 mg dose would be appropriate for Lewis (0.1 mg/kg $\times$ 20 kg = 2 mg). Meperidine would be initiated at $\sim$ 1 mg/kg per dose.

15d. (B) Since Lewis is receiving intravenous fats, it would be prudent to obtain a baseline triglyceride concentration with subsequent concentrations monitored based on initial lab value, change in lipid dose, and duration of therapy.

15e. (B) The estimated daily caloric requirements for pediatric patients are as follows: preterm infants 85–130 kcal/kg, infants 90–100 kcal/kg, ages 1–7 y/o 75–90 kcal/kg, ages 7–12 y/o 60–75 kcal/kg, and by 18 y/o 30-60 kcal/kg.

15f. (A) Peripheral parenteral nutrition solutions consists of low concentrations of dextrose and amino acids, and therefore large volumes are often needed to meet nutrient requirements. They are intended for short term use with phlebitis being the most common complication. To reduce the incidence of phlebitis, it is recommended for the solution's osmolarity not to exceed 600 mOsm/L; however, higher osmolarities may be tolerated for short periods. Infusing lipids simultaneously with the dextrose and amino acid solution will reduce the solution's osmolarity.

15g. (B) Hyperglycemia is the most common metabolic complication of total parenteral nutrition and may be a result of infusing the solution too rapidly or the inability of the pancreas to increase endogenous insulin. Insulin therapy may be necessary to maintain desired serum glucose concentrations.

15h. (A) Travasol is an amino acid preparation commonly used in pediatric and adult patients. Trophamine is an amino acid preparation specifically formulated to meet the needs of neonatal patients. Hepatamine and Nephramine are formulated for patients with hepatic or renal dysfunction, respectively.

15i. (B) Each gram of dextrose contributes 5 mOsm/L. A 10% dextrose solution contains 10 grams/100 mL or 100 grams/L. Therefore, if 1 gram = 5 mOsm, then 100 grams = 500 mOsm.

15j. (C) Dextrose provides 3.4 kcal/gram. A 10% dextrose solution provides 10 grams/100 mL. Since the TPN is infusing at 55 mLs/hr, Lewis will receive 1320 mLs/day. Therefore, 10 gms /100 mL = x/1320 ml; x = 132 gms/day. So, 3.4 kcal/gram = x/132 grams = 448.8 kcals/day.

15k. (D) TPN at 55 mLs/hr = 1320 mLs/day. A 10% dextrose solution contains 10 gms/100 mL. Therefore 10 gms/100 mL = x/1320 mL; x = 132 gms needed for 24 hours. Dextrose 70% = 70 gms/100 mL, therefore, 70 gms/100ml = 132 gms/x; x = 188.6 mLs of dextrose 70% required.

15l. (B) As a result of issues regarding osmolarity, the maximum recommended concentration of dextrose for a peripheral TPN is typically 12.5%. A 12.5% dextrose solution contributes 625 mOsm/L.

15m. (C) Intravenous lipid 10 and 20% solutions provide 1.1 and 2 kcal/mL, respectively. Lewis is receiving 20% lipids at 17 mLs/hr $\times$ 12 hours. Therefore, the total volume = 17 mLs/hr $\times$ 12 hrs = 204 mL. Therefore, 2 kcal/mL = x/204 mL; x = 408 kcal.

15n. (C) Lewis is receiving sodium as NaCl 6 mEq/L and Na Acetate 24 mEq/L for a total of 30 mEq/L. The total volume infused per day is 55 mL/hr x 24 hrs = 1320 mL. Therefore, 30 mEq Na/1000 mL = x/1320 mL; x = 39.6 mEq Na per day.

15o. (A) Lewis is prescribed 14 mEq/L of potassium phosphate. At a TPN rate of 55 mL/hr $\times$ 24 hr, he receives 1320 mL/day. Therefore, 14 mEq/1000 mL = x / 1320 mL; x = 18.5 mEq/day. Each milliliter of intravenous potassium phosphate contains 4.4 mEq of potassium and 3 mmol of phosphorus. Therefore, 4.4 mEq potassium/3mmol phosphorus = 18.5 mEq potassium/x; x = 12.6 mmol of phosphorus.

15p. (B) Sodium acetate is converted to sodium bicarbonate in-vivo. Since Lewis' serum bicarbonate is moderately elevated, it may be desirable to eliminate exogenous sources of bicarbonate.

15q. (D) PTE-5 is a product that contains the trace elements chromium (1 mcg/mL), copper (0.1 mg/mL), manganese (0.025 mg/mL), selenium (15 mcg/mL), and zinc (1 mg/mL).

CASE 16

16a. (B) Given Samuel's allergy to penicillin, the possibility exists that he may react similarly to a cephalosporin such as cefazolin. The incidence of such a reaction is likely less than 10 % with the incidence being lower for the higher-generation cephalosporins.

16b. (D) Ranitidine (Zantac) is compatible in TPN

solutions. As opposed to intermittent dosing, adding ranitidine to TPN solutions results in cost savings and less nursing time needed for administration.

16c. (C) Antibiotics are commonly prescribed before and after surgical procedures due to the possibility of infections resulting from surgery. The antibiotic chosen is determined by the type of procedure performed.

16d. (C) The pediatric dosage of cefazolin is 50–100 mg/kg/day divided in three doses. The usual adult dose is 1 gram iv q 8 hours. Therefore, a dosage of 1 gram iv q 8 hours would be appropriate for Samuel (1000 mg iv q 8 h = 3000 mg/day; 3000 mg/day divided by 40 kg = 75 mg/kg/day).

16e. (A) Samuel is most likely prescribed ondansetron for nausea and vomiting that might occur after his surgical procedure. Additionally, he is prescribed an opiate (morphine) for pain that might result in nausea and vomiting as well.

16f. (C) An appropriate pediatric dose of ondansetron is 0.15 mg/kg iv q 8 h prn. Therefore, for Samuel, 0.15 mg/kg × 40 kg = 6 mg.

16g. (D) Daily fluid requirements are as follows: 1–10 kg = 100 mL/kg; 10–20 kg = 1000 mL + 50 mL/each kg over 10 kg; > 20 kg = 1500 mL + 20 mL/each kg over 20 kg. Therefore, for a 40-kg patient such as Samuel, his daily fluid requirement is 1500 mL + (20 mL × 20) = 1900 mLs.

16h. (D) "Central" TPN's are administered via central veins, usually via the subclavian or internal jugular vein. Other central lines including Broviac, Hickman's, or PIC lines may also be used. Since the solution's osmolarity is not usually an issue with central lines, highly concentrated solutions may be infused resulting in less fluid being administered. Central lines are preferred to peripheral lines when long term nutritional support is needed.

16i. (D) Samuel's total daily TPN volume is 80 mL/hr × 24 hrs = 1920 mL/day. For a 2.5% amino acid solution, he requires 48 grams of amino acids per day (2.5 grams/100 mL = x/1920 mL; x = 48 grams). Using a 10% amino acid solution to obtain 48 grams; 10 grams/100 mL = 48 grams/x; x = 480 mLs.

16j. (B) Calories from protein are typically not included in the caloric calculation as sufficient nonprotein calories must be provided to meet basal metabolic energy demands, ensure growth and development, and to prevent the use of protein from the parenteral solution, muscle, or visceral protein merely as an energy source.

16k. (B) Parenteral dextrose provides 3.4 kcal/gram.

Since Samuel is receiving 1920 mL of TPN per day of which contains 25% dextrose, he is receiving 480 grams of dextrose per day (25 grams/100 mL = x/1920 mL; x = 480 grams). If one gram of dextrose = 3.4 kcal, then 480 grams = 1632 kcal (1 gram/3.4 kcal = 480 grams/x; x = 1632 kcal).

16l. (D) *Malassezia furfur* is commonly associated with intravenous lipid solutions. When preparing lipids, as with any parenterally administered product, strict aseptic techniques should be used. As a means of quality assessment, it is also prudent to occasionally culture the lipid product remaining in the syringe or container once the patient has received his dose.

16m. (D) Hyperglycemia is a common metabolic effect of total parenteral nutrition. Given Samuel's elevated serum glucose concentration, it would be prudent to begin insulin therapy. Intensive care patients with elevated serum glucose concentrations develop more complications.

16n. (B) Daily serum electrolytes and minerals should be assessed while patients are being stabilized on TPN solutions using the appropriate adjustments. Since Samuel's sodium and chloride serum concentrations are low, the NaCl additive in his TPN should be adjusted.

16o. (D) Calcium and phosphorus will precipitate in TPN solutions if a certain concentration is exceeded. To ensure compatibility, the TPN should not contain more than 60 "units" of calcium and phosphorus when using TrophAmine or 45 "units" when using other amino acid solutions. Up to 75 "units" may be added to TrophAmine containing TPN's if L-cysteine is added to the TPN solution.

16p. (C)

16q. (B)

CASE 17

17a. (C) Schizophrenia does not imply a split personality, but rather is a chronic disorder of thought and affect with the individual having difficulty with interpersonal relationships and an ability to function in society. Although increasing evidence suggests a genetic basis, no abnormality has been isolated. It most commonly occurs in late adolescence or early adulthood with the onset tending to be earlier in males.

17b. (D) Schizophrenia symptoms are typically classified as "positive" or "negative." Positive symptoms include hallucinations and delusions, whereas negative symptoms include affective flattening, alogia, anhedonia, and avolition.

17c. (B) The atypical antipsychotic agents improve both positive and negative symptoms associated with schizophrenia. These include clozapine, risperidone, olanzapine, and quetiapine.

17d. (E) Although blockade of dopamine and serotonin receptors is commonly associated with antipsychotic agents, they also block others including histamine, muscarinic, and α-adrenergic receptors.

17e. (A) Haloperidol is classified as a high potency traditional or typical antipsychotic agent.

17f. (B) Extrapyramidal side effects are more commonly associated with high potency typical antipsychotic agents. Sedation, orthostasis, and anticholinergic effects tend to occur more commonly with low potency agents.

17g. (D) Like risperidone, Olanzapine(Zyprexa) is an atypical antipsychotic agent.

17h. (A) Binding to the dopamine (D_2) receptor is associated with the occurrence of extrapyramidal side effects. Compared with the typical agents, atypical agents have a lower affinity for these receptors, and thus result in a lower incidence of such adverse effects.

17i. (D) Among the atypical agents, quetiapine has the lowest D_2 binding and thus the lowest incidence of extrapyramidal adverse effects.

17j. (D) Tardive dyskinesia is a syndrome of abnormal involuntary movements typically described as a buccolingual–masticatory syndrome or orofacial movements. It usually occurs after many months to years of treatment and may be irreversible, despite discontinuation of the antipsychotic agent.

17k. (B) Several classes of medications are used to treat the extrapyramidal side effects of antipsychotic agents. These include antimuscarinics, antihistamines, dopamine agonists, benzodiazepines, and β-adrenergic blockers. Benztropine is an antimuscarinic agent used to provide relief from extrapyramidal adverse effects.

17l. (B) Although not FDA approved for intravenous use, multiple studies have proven the safety and efficacy of intravenous haloperidol for the treatment of agitated patients. The lactate formulation should be used as the decanoate formulation is a long-acting preparation that is administered monthly and only via the intramuscular route. For Lee, the recommended adult dose of 2–5 mg would be appropriate.

17m. (D) Risperidone (Risperdal) is available for oral administration as tablets and an oral solution. The oral solution is not compatible with cola or tea.

17n. (C) The recommended dosage titration for adult patients is 1 mg po bid on day 1, 2 mg po bid on day 2, and 3 mg po bid on day 3. Doses in excess of 6 mg/day may result in a higher incidence of extrapyramidal side effects because of an increased affinity for D_2 receptors without increased efficacy. The safety of doses > 16 mg/day has not been established.

17o. (D) The typical initial dose of lorazepam is 0.05–0.1 mg/kg with a maximum single dose of 4 mg.

CASE 18

18a. (E) Diagnostic criteria for nephrotic syndrome includes generalized edema, hypoproteinemia (albumin < 2 g/dL), proteinuria (24-hour urine protein > 50 mg/kg), and hypercholesterolemia (200 mg/dL).

18b. (E) Complications associated with nephrotic syndrome include scrotal edema, pulmonary edema, oliguria, infections, thromboembolisms, hyperlipidemia, and impaired growth.

18c. (B) The reduced serum albumin concentration in nephrotic syndrome patients results in a significant reduction in plasma oncotic pressure. Therefore, circulatory volume is mobilized to the interstitial spaces resulting in generalized edema.

18d. (B) Intravenous albumin is effective in mobilizing fluid into the vascular space. The rate of increase in the oncotic pressure is directly proportional to the rate of expansion of the intravascular volume.

18e. (A) Depending on the volume output and the degree of edema, furosemide (Lasix) is often given with or after the dose of albumin.

18f. (D) Albumin 5% = 5 gms/100 mL; therefore, 5 gms/100 mL = 12.5 gms/x; x = 250 mLs.

18g. (C) The albumin regimen for the treatment of nephrotic syndrome is albumin 25%, 1 gm/kg. Therefore, the dose for Carrie would be 13 grams (1 gm/kg × 13 kg = 13 gms) of 25% albumin. Since 25% albumin is available in 50 mL bottles, one bottle provides 12.5 gm of albumin (25 gms/100 mL = 12.5 gms/50 mLs). Therefore, Carrie should receive 50 mLs of 25% albumin or 12.5 gms as opposed 13 gms that would require opening a second bottle of albumin.

18h. (B) In the event Carrie is allergic to sulfur,

ethacrynic acid (Edecrin), a loop diuretic that is devoid of sulfur, should be prescribed.

18i. (A) As the intravascular volume is expanded with the administration of albumin, renal perfusion improves at which time the opportunity to reduce accumulated fluid occurs. Furosemide inhibits active reabsorption of chloride in the ascending loop of Henle resulting in urinary excretion of sodium, chloride, and water. The furosemide is dosed at 1–2 mg/kg intravenously.

18j. (C) For the treatment of nephrotic syndrome, prednisone is typically dosed at 60 mg/m² or 2 mg/kg daily. Therefore, for Carrie, 2 mg/kg × 13 kg = 26 mg. If prednisone tablets are used, for convenience of dosing, 25 mg should be prescribed as the tablets are available in 5- and 20-mg strengths.

18k. (E) For steroid-resistant nephrotic syndrome or continued proteinuria, alternative agents including cyclosporine, cyclophosphamide, chlorambucil, levamisole, angiotensin converting enzyme inhibitors, mizoribine, mycophenolate mofetil, and nonsteroidal antiinflammatory agents have been prescribed. Cyclophosphamide and chlorambucil have been used most commonly. Of note, their side effect profiles are the major reason for their use as alternative therapies.

18l. (A) As is lansoprazole (Prevacid), Protonix (pantoprazole) is a proton pump inhibitor.

18m. (B) The initial daily pediatric dose of lansoprazole is 15 mg for patients < 30 kg and 30 mg for patients > 30 kg. Therefore, the correct dose for Carrie (13 kg) would be 15 mg po qd.

Pediatric Out-Patient

*It is better to lead by example
than by fear*

This section consists of 18 prescriptions followed by corresponding retail pharmacy patient profiles representing pharmacotherapy prescribed to outpatients. The profiles only include information for the most recently filled prescription for each medication listed. Each patient profile is followed by multiple-choice questions pertaining to the prescription and profile information. Choose the one best-lettered response for each item. The correct answers are provided at the end of this section. The reader is encouraged to attempt all questions for each case or for the entire section before referring to the answer key. Moreover, where appropriate, the answer key provides an explanation of the correct response and should serve as an additional learning tool for the reader.

CASE 1

John Henderson, MD
234 Parkway Drive
Naples, FL 33323

Patient: Beverly Jones

Date: September 23, 2002

Amoxil 125 mg/5 mL
75 mLs
1 tsp po tid × 7 days

Refill: None

Doctor: John Henderson

PHARMACY PROFILE

Patient: Beverly Jones

Patient Weight: 10 kg   **Age:** 13 m/o

Medical History: Otitis media

Allergies: None

Medication Profile:

Date	Medication	Quantity
07/11/02	Augmentin 125 mg po tid	150 mLs

1a. Which of the following best describes acute otitis media?

   A. A red tympanic membrane without middle ear fluid
   B. Middle ear fluid accompanied by a sign of infection
   C. Middle ear fluid in the absence of a sign of infection
   D. Inflammation of the middle ear

1b. Which of the following is true regarding otitis media?

   A. Usually follows a viral infection of the nasopharynx
   B. Most common reason for prescribing antibiotics to children
   C. Typically occurs more commonly in females
   D. A and B only
   E. A, B, and C

1c. Which of the following is a risk factor for otitis media?

   A. Day care attendance
   B. Passive exposure to cigarette smoke
   C. Lack of breast feeding
   D. A and B only
   E. A, B, and C

1d. The most common bacterial pathogen associated with otitis media is _____.

   A. *H. influenzae*
   B. *M. catarrhalis*
   C. *S. pneumoniae*
   D. *E. coli*

1e. Which of the following was Beverly prescribed in July, 2002?

A. Ampicillin and sulbactam
B. Ampicillin and potassium clavulanate
C. Amoxicillin and sulbactam
D. Amoxicillin and potassium clavulanate

1f. Which of the following is most similar to sulbactam and potassium clavulanate?

A. Ticarcillin
B. Tazobactam
C. Sulfamethoxazole
D. Imipenem

1g. Which of the following is the most common adverse effect associated with Augmentin therapy?

A. Nausea
B. Diarrhea
C. Rash
D. Serum Sickness

1h. If Augmentin 125 mg/5 mL was dispensed for Beverly's previous prescription, 150 mLs would have provided her with how many days of therapy?

A. 5
B. 7
C. 10
D. 15

1i. Which of the following is true of Augmentin 250- and 500-mg tablets?

A. They should always be administered with food
B. Two 250-mg tablets are equivalent to one 500-mg tablet
C. The dose is based on the antibiotic component of the product
D. B and C only
E. A, B, and C

1j. The drug of choice for the treatment of acute otitis media is _____.

A. Amoxil
B. Augmentin
C. Rocephin
D. Zithromax

1k. Approximately how many milliliters of Amoxil should have been prescribed to Beverly?

A. 75 mL
B. 100 mL
C. 125 mL
D. 150 mL

1l. Which of the following counseling tips should Beverly's mother receive regarding her child's amoxicillin therapy?

A. Shake the amoxicillin bottle prior to use
B. After completing 7 days of therapy, discard any remaining medication
C. May discontinue therapy in 3 days if Beverly is no longer febrile
D. A and B only
E. A, B, and C

1m. A more appropriate amoxicillin dose for Beverly would be _____.

A. 250 mg po bid
B. 250 mg po tid
C. 450 mg po bid
D. 450 mg po tid

1n. The most likely reason for adjusting Beverly's amoxicillin dose is to provide increased activity against _____.

A. β-lactamase producing bacteria
B. β-lactamase producing *M. catarrhalis*
C. resistant *H. influenzae*
D. resistant *S. pneumoniae*

1o. Which of the following is an alternative therapy for otitis media for potentially noncompliant patients?

A. Zithromax
B. Rocephin
C. Septra DS
D. A and B only
E. A, B, and C

CASE 2

Steve Holmes, MD
101 Briar Drive
Raleigh, NC 27866

Patient: Todd Stevens

Date: July 14, 2002

Advair 100/50
#1
2 puffs qid

Refill: 6

Doctor: Steve Holmes

PHARMACY PROFILE

Patient: Todd Stevens

Patient Weight: 50 kg   **Age:** 12 y/o

Medical History: Asthma

Allergies: None

Medication Profile:

Date	Medication	Quantity
1/30/02	Ventolin 2 puffs prn	1
1/30/02	Vanceril DS 2 puffs bid	1

2a. The active ingredient in Ventolin is

_____.

A. Levalbuterol
B. Albuterol
C. Salmeterol
D. Isoproterenol

2b. The active ingredient of Ventolin is classified as a(n) _____.

A. anticholinergic agent
B. mast-cell stabilizer
C. vorticosteroid
D. β-agonist

2c. Each actuation of Ventolin delivers _____ of active drug.

A. 45 mcg
B. 45 mg
C. 90 mcg
D. 90 mg

2d. Which of the following adverse effects is associated with Ventolin?

A. Tachycardia
B. Restlessness
C. Hypokalemia
D. A and B only
E. A, B, and C

2e. Ventolin is available in which of the following dosage forms?

A. Tablets
B. Solution for inhalation
C. Capsules for inhalation
D. A and B only
E. A, B, and C

2f. The active ingredient in Vanceril DS is _____.

A. fluticasone
B. budesonide
C. flunisolide
D. beclomethasone

2g. Vanceril is classified as a(n) _____.

    A. corticosteroid
    B. β-agonist
    C. anticholinergic agent
    D. leukotriene antagonist

2h. Each prescribed dose of Vanceril DS provides Todd with _____ mcg of active medication.

    A. 21
    B. 42
    C. 84
    D. 168

2i. Which of the following adverse effects is Todd most likely to encounter from his Vanceril DS therapy?

    A. Adrenal suppression
    B. Growth retardation
    C. Hoarseness
    D. B and C only
    E. A, B, and C

2j. Which of the following medications is most similar to Vanceril DS?

    A. Singulair
    B. Zyflo
    C. AeroBid
    D. Intal

2k. In the past, Todd inquired if he used his Vanceril DS and Ventolin inhalers at the same time, which one should he inhale first? Which of the following statements would be the most appropriate response to his inquiry?

    A. The inhalers should never be used within 30 minutes of each other
    B. The Vanceril DS should be dosed first
    C. The Ventolin should be dosed first
    D. The order in which they are used is irrelevant

2l. Advair is a combination product that contains _____ and _____.

    A. beclomethasone, salmeterol
    B. fluticasone, salmeterol
    C. beclomethasone, albuterol
    D. fluticasone, albuterol

2m. Which of the following statements is true of Advair?

    A. Is indicated for the treatment of acute bronchospasms
    B. Is available in three different doses with the quantity of the β-agonist component varying between the different preparations
    C. Is only available as a Diskus dosage form
    D. A and B only
    E. A, B, and C

2n. Of the following medications, which would be most appropriate to prescribe concurrently with Advair?

    A. Albuterol
    B. Beclomethasone
    C. Salmeterol
    D. Ipratropium bromide

2o. Todd's Advair dose should be adjusted to _____.

    A. 2 puffs qd
    B. 1 puff bid
    C. 2 puffs bid
    D. 1 puff tid

CASE 3

Sam Elliott, MD
831 Peach Street
Atlanta, GA 26788

Patient: Tracy Heights

Date: March 14, 2002

Albuterol 0.083% inhalation solution
#25
2.5 mg neb prn exacerbations

Refill: 2

Doctor: Sam Elliott

PHARMACY PROFILE

Patient: Tracy Heights

Patient Weight: 35 kg   **Age:** 12 y/o

Medical History: Asthma

Allergies: Peanuts

Medication Profile:

Date	Medication	Quantity
02/15/02	Xopenex 2.5 mg nebs prn	30
02/15/02	Flovent 44 mcg inh	1
02/15/02	Singulair 5 mg qid	120 tablets

3a. The active ingredient in Xopenex is _____.

   A. Racemic albuterol
   B. Levalbuterol
   C. Dextroalbuterol
   D. Salmeterol

3b. Xopenex is classified as a(n) _____.

   A. anticholinergic agent
   B. rapid acting β-2 agonist
   C. long acting β-2 agonist
   D. leukotriene antagonist

3c. A more appropriate dose of Xopenex for Tracy is
   _____.

   A. 0.31 mcg
   B. 0.31 mg
   C. 0.63 mcg
   D. 0.63 mg

3d. Xopenex is available in which of the following dosage forms?

   A. Metered dose inhaler
   B. Inhalation solution
   C. Diskus inhaler
   D. A and B only
   E. A, B, and C

3e. The active ingredient in Singulair is _____.

   A. zafirlukast
   B. montelukast
   C. zileuton
   D. palivizumab

3f. Singulair is classified as a _____.

   A. corticosteroid
   B. leukotriene antagonist
   C. long active β-2 agonist
   D. mast-cell stabilizer

3g. Which of the following is true of Singulair?

A. Dosage adjustments are necessary in the presence of renal dysfunction
B. The tablets should be swallowed whole and not crushed or chewed
C. Is extensively metabolized by the liver
D. A and B only
E. A, B, and C

3h. Compared with other medications in its same class, an advantage of Singulair includes _____.

A. Less frequent dosing
B. Pediatric dosing guidelines
C. Less liver toxicity
D. A and B only
E. A, B, and C

3i. The correct dosage of Singulair for Tracy is _____.

A. 4 mg po qd
B. 4 mg po bid
C. 5 mg po qd
D. 10 mg po qd

3j. The active ingredient in Flovent is _____.

A. flunisolide
B. budesonide
C. triamcinolone
D. fluticasone

3k. Tracy's Flovent should be administered _____ a day.

A. Once
B. Twice
C. Three times
D. Four times

3l. How many milliliters of the albuterol solution are needed to provide Tracy with her prescribed dose?

A. 0.5 mL
B. 1 mL
C. 2 mL
D. 3 mL

3m. Which of the following statements is true regarding Tracy's albuterol prescription?

A. Should not be filled since she is receiving a similar drug that is less expensive
B. Should not be filled since she is receiving a similar drug that is more effective
C. Should not be filled since she is receiving a similar drug that produces less adverse effects
D. Should be filled, and the similar drug that she is receiving should be discontinued

3n. Frequent albuterol refills should alert the pharmacist to recommend which of the following to Tracy's physician?

A. Her asthma is becoming progressively worse
B. Her controller medications should be adjusted
C. The albuterol dose should be increased to 5 mg
D. A and B only
E. A, B, and C

CASE 4

Thomas Beck, MD
1150 Bird Drive
Charlotte, NC 28976

Patient: Gary Anderson

Date: January 26, 2002

Zithromax 100 mg/5 mL
100 mg × 1, then 50 mg qd × 4 days

Refill: None

Doctor: Thomas Beck

PHARMACY PROFILE

Patient: Gary Anderson

Patient Weight: 10 kg   **Age:** 13 m/o

Medical History: Otitis media (noncompliant with meds), Received IPV, MMR, Varicella, and *Pneumococcal* vaccines at 12 months of age

Allergies: Sulfur

Medication Profile:

Date	Medication	Quantity
01/03/02	Amoxil 125 mg tid	150 mL

4a. How many milliliters of azithromycin should be dispensed to Gary?

A. 15 mL
B. 30 mL
C. 45 mL
D. 60 mL

4b. Which of the following would serve as alternative azithromycin regimens for Gary?

A. 300 mg po × 1 dose
B. 100 mg po qd × 3 days
C. 50 mg po qd × 5 days
D. A and B only
E. A, B, and C

4c. Which of the following medications would be most appropriate to prescribe for the treatment of resistant otitis media in a noncompliant patient?

A. Cefotaxime
B. Ceftriaxone
C. Cefazolin
D. Cefuroxime

4d. IPV refers to _____ polio vaccine.

A. intermediate
B. inactivated
C. immunological
D. inferior

4e. How many doses of IPV should Gary have received prior to the dose noted on his medication profile?

A. 0
B. 1
C. 2
D. 3

4f. Gary's next dose of measles, mumps, and rubella (MMR) vaccine should be given at age _____ years.

A. 2–4
B. 4–6
C. 6–8
D. 8–10

4g. Which of the following is true regarding the MMR vaccine?

A. Is a live vaccine
B. A total of 3 doses is recommended for children
C. Is associated with an increase in autism
D. A and B only
E. A, B, and C

4h. Which of the following is the appropriate dose and route for the MMR vaccine?

A. 0.5 mL, SC
B. 0.5 mL, IM
C. 1 mL, SC
D. 1 mL, IM

4i. If not given simultaneously, MMR and varicella vaccines should be separated by at least _____ days.

A. 30
B. 45
C. 60
D. 90

4j. The brand name for the varicella vaccine is

_____.

A. Valcyte
B. Varivax
C. Valtrex
D. Virazole

4k. Which of the following is true concerning the varicella vaccine?

A. Two doses are recommended for patients ≥ 13 months
B. Salicylates should not be used for 6 weeks after vaccination with varicella vaccine
C. The preferred route of administration is intramuscular (IM)
D. A and B only
E. A, B, and C

4l. How many doses of *pneumococcal* vaccine should Gary have received prior to his 12-month dose?

A. 1
B. 2
C. 3
D. 4

4m. Which of the following is the trade name for the *pneumococcal* vaccine administered to Gary?

A. Pneumovax 23
B. Pnu-Imune 23
C. Prevnar
D. Pepcid

4n. Which of the following is the recommended dose and route for the *pneumococcal* vaccine for children?

A. 0.5 mL, SC
B. 0.5 mL, IM
C. 1 mL SC
D. 1 mL, IM

4o. Which of the following is true of the *pneumococcal* vaccine prescribed to Gary?

A. It is a hexavalent vaccine
B. The first dose is usually administered at 2 months of age
C. Should not be administered to immunocompromised patients
D. The last dose is recommended at 4–6 years of age

4p. Which of the following immunizations is contraindicated in patients with a known anaphylactic reaction to neomycin?

A. IPV
B. Varicella
C. Pneumococcal
D. A and B only
E. A, B, and C

CASE 5

Rick Hayes, MD
101 Cedar Street
Mayberry, NC 56767

Patient: Bonnie Rhimes

Date: March 14, 2002

Fluoride Ion 0.25 mg/drop
1 bottle
1 mL qd

Refill: 6

Doctor: Rick Hayes

PHARMACY PROFILE

Patient: Bonnie Rhimes

Patient Weight: 7 kg   **Age:** 7 m/o

Medical History: Received DTaP, Hib, and Hep B vaccines at 6 months of age

Allergies: None

Medication Profile:

Date	Medication	Quantity

5a. Which of the following is a fluoride product?

  A. Flura-Drops
  B. Luride
  C. Gel Kam
  D. A and B only
  E. A, B, and C

5b. A more appropriate dose of fluoride for Bonnie is
  _____.

  A. 1 drop
  B. 2 drops
  C. 0.25 mL
  D. 0.5 mL

5c. Which of the following vaccines was most likely given to Bonnie soon after birth?

  A. Hepatitis B
  B. DTaP
  C. Hib
  D. PCV

5d. Which component of the DTaP vaccine is predominantly associated with neurological complications?

  A. Diphtheria
  B. Tetanus
  C. Pertussis
  D. Polio

5e. Which of the following is a contraindication to receiving the DTaP vaccine?

  A. Encephalopathy within 7 days of the vaccine
  B. A seizure within 3 days of the vaccine
  C. Shock-like state within 48 hours of vaccine
  D. A and B only
  E. A, B, and C

5f. Which of the following is the correct dose and route of administration for the DTaP immunization?

  A. 0.5 mL, IM
  B. 0.5 mL, SC
  C. 1 mL, IM
  D. 1 mL, SC

5g. In providing the five scheduled doses of pertussis, _____ doses of acellular pertussis are recommended.

A. 2
B. 3
C. 4
D. 5

5h. Vaccination against tetanus and diphtheria (Td) should be given at 11 to 15 years of age and should continue throughout life at _____ year intervals.

A. 5
B. 10
C. 15
D. 20

5i. Bonnie should have also received a dose of *Haemophilus influenzae* type-b conjugate vaccine at _____ month(s) of age.

A. 1
B. 2
C. 4
D. B and C only
E. A, B, and C

5j. If PedvaxHIB had been dosed at each scheduled visit to immunize Bonnie, the scheduled dose at _____ months of age would not have been required.

A. 1
B. 2
C. 4
D. 6

5k. Which of the following is a *H. influenzae* type-b immunization product?

A. HibTiter
B. ProHibit
C. Comvax
D. A and B only
E. A, B, and C

5l. Provided Bonnie's 6-month hepatitis B vaccine completed her series, how many doses should she have received before her 6-month dose?

A. 1
B. 2
C. 3
D. 4

5m. Which of the following products contains hepatitis-B vaccine?

A. Recombivax HB
B. Engerix
C. Havrix
D. A and B only
E. A, B, and C

5n. If Bonnie had been born to a HbsAg-positive mother, she should have received hepatitis B immune globulin within _____ hours of birth.

A. 6
B. 12
C. 18
D. 24

5o. At 12 months of age, Bonnie is noted to have contracted HIV from a blood transfusion. Her current CD4 cell percentage is > 25%. Which of the following 12-month immunizations may Bonnie receive?

A. Varicella
B. MMR
C. PCV
D. A and B only
E. A, B, and C

CASE 6

Steve Woldendorf, MD
945 Clay Court
Chapel Hill, NC 27599

Patient: Sarah Murray

Date: December 10, 2002

Lasix 10 mg/mL solution
20 mL
Give 0.25 mL po bid

Refill: None

Doctor: Steve Woldendorf

PHARMACY PROFILE

Patient: Sarah Murray

Patient Weight: 5 kg   **Age:** 6 m/o

Medical History: 36-weeks gestation, BPD,
received palivizumab on 11/01/02

Allergies: None

Medication Profile:

Date	Medication	Quantity
11/18/02	Albuterol nebs 1 mg q 6 h prn	25
11/18/02	Dexamethasone 0.5 mg qd	30

6a. How many milliliters of furosemide are needed to provide Sarah with a 30-day supply as prescribed?

A. 10 mL
B. 15 mL
C. 20 mL
D. 25 mL

6b. How many milligrams of furosemide is Sarah prescribed per day?

A. 0.25 mg
B. 0.5 mg
C. 2.5 mg
D. 5 mg

6c. Which of the following is true regarding palivizumab?

A. Is a monoclonal antibody
B. Is indicated for the treatment of RSV
C. Should not be administered with live vaccines
D. A and B only
E. A, B, and C

6d. The name brand for palivizumab is _____.

A. Synercid
B. Synagis
C. Synalar
D. Synacort

6e. Which of the following dates would be most appropriate to administer Sarah's next dose of palivizumab?

   A. November 15, 2002
   B. December 1, 2002
   C. December 15, 2002
   D. January 1, 2003

6f. The correct dose of palivizumab for Sarah is _____ milligrams.

   A. 75
   B. 500
   C. 1250
   D. 3750

6g. Which of the following is the recommended route of administration for palivizumab?

   A. PO
   B. SC
   C. IM
   D. IV

6h. The trade name for respiratory syncytial virus immune globulin (RSV-IVIG) is _____.

   A. Virazole
   B. RespiGam
   C. Synagis
   D. Gamimune N

6i. Had Sarah been treated with RSV-IVIG in lieu of palivizumab, the correct dose of RSV-IVIG for her would have been _____ milligrams.

   A. 75
   B. 500
   C. 1250
   D. 3750

6j. Which of the following is true regarding the administration of RSV-IVIG?

   A. MMR vaccine may be given concurrently with RSV-IVIG
   B. It is administered via IM injection
   C. There is a risk of transmission of blood-borne pathogens
   D. The solution should be shaken well prior to administration

6k. After entry into the vial, the dose of RSV-IVIG should be initiated within _____ hours.

   A. 6
   B. 8
   C. 10
   D. 12

CASE 7

Sam Mahoney, MD
768 Professional Drive
Los Angeles, CA 90036

Patient: <u>Peter Parker</u>   **Date:** <u>April 15, 2002</u>

Concerta 36 mg
60
1 tablet bid

Doctor: <u>Sam Mahoney</u>
Refill: <u>0</u>   DEA # <u>1234563</u>

PHARMACY PROFILE

Patient: Peter Parker   **Patient Weight:** 30 kg   **Age:** 6 y/o

Medical History: ADHD   **Allergies:** None

Medication Profile:

Date	Medication	Quantity
03/17/02	Ritalin 5 mg po tid	90

7a. Which of the following is true of attention deficit hyperactivity disorder?

   A. For proper diagnosis, the onset of symptoms should occur before age 7
   B. Is characterized by inattention, impulsivity, and hyperactivity
   C. Occurs throughout life in some individuals
   D. A and B only
   E. A, B, and C

7b. In the treatment of attention deficit hyperactivity disorder, Ritalin is believed to act through blocking the reuptake of which of the following neurotransmitters?

   A. Dopamine
   B. Norepinephrine
   C. Epinephrine
   D. A and B only
   E. A, B, and C

7c. The duration of action of Ritalin is approximately _____ hours.

   A. 3–4
   B. 4–6
   C. 6–8
   D. 8–10

7d. Which of the following is a typical side effect of Ritalin?

   A. Anorexia
   B. Depression
   C. Drowsiness
   D. Convulsions

7e. Which of the following times would be most appropriate to dose Peter's Ritalin?

   A. 6 AM, 12 PM, 4 PM
   B. 6 AM, 12 PM, 9 PM
   C. 9 AM, 3 PM, 9 PM
   D. 9 AM, 12 PM, 6 PM

7f. The maximum recommended daily dose of Ritalin is _____ milligrams.

   A. 20
   B. 40
   C. 60
   D. 80

7g. Which of the following best describes Concerta?

   A. Immediate release methylphenidate
   B. Extended release methylphenidate
   C. Immediate release dexmethylphenidate
   D. Extended release dexmethylphenidate

7h. A more appropriate dosage of Concerta for Peter is _____.

   A. 18 mg po qd
   B. 18 mg po bid
   C. 36 mg po qd
   D. 54 mg po qd

7i. The maximum recommended daily dose of Concerta is _____ milligrams.

   A. 18
   B. 36
   C. 54
   D. 72

7j. Which of the following is a potential contraindication to Concerta therapy?

   A. Tourette's syndrome
   B. Glaucoma
   C. Marked anxiety
   D. A and B only
   E. A, B, and C

CASE 8

William Hacker, MD
900 Doctors Lane
St. Louis, MO 45673

Patient: Robert Jordon

Date: March 27, 2003

Imipramine 25 mg
#60
1 tablet bid

Refill: None

Doctor: William Hacker

PHARMACY PROFILE

Patient: Robert Jordon

Patient Weight: 25 kg   **Age:** 8 y/o

Medical History: ADHD (not well controlled), depression

Allergies: None

Medication Profile:

Date	Medication	Quantity
11/23/02	Adderall 5 mg bid	60
01/15/03	Focalin 5 mg qd	60

8a. Which of the following is a component of Adderall?

   A. d-amphetamine saccharate
   B. d, l-amphetamine aspartate monohydrate
   C. d-amphetamine sulfate
   D. A and B only
   E. A, B, and C

8b. In the event Robert's Adderall had been switched to Adderall XR, an appropriate initial regimen would have been _____.

   A. 5 mg qd
   B. 10 mg qd
   C. 15 mg qd
   D. 20 mg qd

8c. The maximum recommended dose of Adderall XR is _____ milligrams.

   A. 20
   B. 30
   C. 40
   D. 60

8d. Which of the following is the active component of Focalin?

   A. Dexmethylphenidate
   B. L-methylphenidate
   C. Dexamphetamine
   D. L-amphetamine

8e. An appropriate initial regimen of Focalin for Robert would have been _____.

    A. 2.5 mg po bid
    B. 5 mg po bid
    C. 7.5 mg po bid
    D. 10 mg po bid

8f. In the treatment of ADHD, which of the following medications has the longest duration of action?

    A. Ritalin LA
    B. Concerta
    C. Metadate ER
    D. Focalin

8g. Which of the following medications is associated with hepatotoxicity?

    A. Focalin
    B. Adderall
    C. Cylert
    D. Tofranil

8h. Which of the following is the most likely reason Robert is prescribed imipramine?

    A. The maximum dose of Adderall had been used
    B. The maximum dose of Focalin had been prescribed
    C. Antidepressants are more effective than stimulants for the treatment of ADHD
    D. Robert was recently diagnosed with depression

8i. Which of the following is a possible side effect from imipramine therapy?

    A. Insomnia
    B. Blurred vision
    C. Polyuria
    D. Hypertension

8j. The brand name for imipramine is _____.

    A. Tofranil
    B. Elavil
    C. Norpramin
    D. Sinequan

8k. Which of the following therapies for ADHD would most likely increase the incidence of seizure activity?

    A. Concerta
    B. Cylert
    C. Buspar
    D. Wellbutrin

8l. Which of the following is a non-stimulant drug indicated for the treatment of ADHD?

    A. Atomoxetine
    B. Pemoline
    C. Dexamphetamine
    D. Dexmethylphenidate

CASE 9

Bert Anderson, MD
900 Center Drive
Charlotte, NC 25689

Patient: Samantha Roberts

Date: January 17, 2003

Topamax 15 mg
60

Refill: None

Doctor: Bert Anderson

PHARMACY PROFILE

Patient: Samantha Roberts

Patient Weight: 30 kg   **Age:** 8 y/o

Medical History: Epilepsy, frequent seizures

Allergies: Penicillin

Medication Profile:

Date	Medication	Quantity
12/18/02	Dilantin 300 mg po tid	90

9a. Which of the following is an example of a generalized seizure?

   A. Tonic-clonic
   B. Myoclonic
   C. Absence
   D. A and B only
   E. A, B, and C

9b. Which of the following is an inhibitory neurotransmitter?

   A. Acetylcholine
   B. Norepinephrine
   C. Aspartate
   D. γ-aminobutyric acid

9c. Which of the following products contains 92% phenytoin?

   A. Dilantin injection
   B. Dilantin chewable tablets
   C. Dilantin oral suspension
   D. Mesantoin tablets

9d. Which of the following best describes the mechanism of action of Dilantin?

   A. Blockade of sodium channels
   B. Reducing voltage-dependent calcium conductance
   C. Enhancing γ-aminobutyric acid activity
   D. Attenuates activation of glutamate receptors

9e. A reasonable targeted phenytoin serum concentration for Samantha would be

   _____.

   A. 4–12 mcg/mL
   B. 10–20 mcg/mL
   C. 15–40 mcg/mL
   D. 50–100 mcg/mL

9f. Which of the following is an adverse effect associated with phenytoin therapy?

   A. Ataxia
   B. Coarsening of facial features
   C. Gingival hyperplasia
   D. A and B only
   E. A, B, and C

9g. A more appropriate regimen of Dilantin for Samantha would be _____.

A. 25 mg po tid
B. 50 mg po tid
C. 100 mg po tid
D. 150 mg po bid

9h. The active ingredient of Topamax is _____.

A. tiagabine
B. topiramate
C. tolectin
D. torsemide

9i. Topamax is indicated as adjunctive therapy for the treatment of _____.

A. partial seizures
B. tonic-clonic seizures
C. Lennox-Gastaut Syndrome
D. A and B only
E. A, B, and C

9j. Topamax is available in which of the following dosage forms?

A. Tablets
B. Sprinkle capsules
C. Oral solution
D. A and B only
E. A, B, and C

9k. Which of the following is a potential adverse effect associated with Topamax therapy?

A. Insomnia
B. Weight gain
C. Decreased insulin effect
D. Renal calculi

9l. The appropriate "sig" for Samantha's Topamax would be "one cap po _____."

A. qd
B. bid
C. tid
D. qid

9m. Prescribing Topamax concurrently with Dilantin in Samantha may result in _____ serum concentrations.

A. increased Dilantin
B. decreased Dilantin
C. decreased Topamax
D. A and C only
E. B and C only

CASE 10

David Hawkins, MD
900 Faye Drive
Garner, NC 27527

Patient: Faith Edwards

Date: May 28, 2003

Lamictal 5 mg tabs
28
1 tab po tid × 2 weeks

Refill: 2

Doctor: David Hawkins

PHARMACY PROFILE

Patient: Faith Edwards

Patient Weight: 25 kg   **Age:** 6 y/o

Medical History: Lennox-Gastaut syndrome

Allergies: None

Medication Profile:

Date	Medication	Quantity
4/17/03	Valproic Acid 500 mg po tid	90
4/17/03	Carnitine 250 mg po bid	90

10a. Which of the following is an injectable product containing valproic acid?

- A. Depakene
- B. Depakote
- C. Depacon
- D. Decadron

10b. Valproic acid has proven efficacy against which of the following seizure types?

- A. Partial
- B. Tonic-clonic
- C. Lennox-Gastaut
- D. A and B only
- E. A, B, and C

10c. Which of the following is a potential adverse effect of valproic acid therapy?

- A. Gastric irritation
- B. Weight gain
- C. Pancreatitis
- D. A and B only
- E. A, B, and C

10d. For patients receiving valproic acid therapy, which of the following laboratory values warrants occasional monitoring?

- A. Liver function tests
- B. Ammonia
- C. Serum creatinine
- D. A and B only
- E. A, B, and C

10e. Which of the following is an accepted therapeutic serum concentration for valproic acid?

    A. 4–12 mcg/mL
    B. 15–40 mcg/mL
    C. 10–20 mg/L
    D. 50–100 mg/L

10f. Faith was most likely prescribed carnitine because _____.

    A. it has anticonvulsant effects
    B. it increases the bioavailability of valproic acid
    C. valproic acid therapy may decrease serum carnitine concentrations
    D. it decreases the progression of Lennox-Gastaut syndrome

10g. A more appropriate dose of carnitine for Faith would be _____.

    A. 500 mg po qd
    B. 500 mg po bid
    C. 500 mg po tid
    D. 500 mg po qid

10h. Lamictal is available in which of the following dosage forms?

    A. Tablets
    B. Capsules
    C. Extended release tablets
    D. A and B only
    E. A, B, and C

10i. Which of the following adverse effects of lamotrigine therapy is most concerning?

    A. Pneumonia
    B. Rash
    C. Hemorrhage
    D. Impaired Vision

10j. A more appropriate regimen of Lamictal for Faith is _____.

    A. 2 mg po qd
    B. 2 mg po bid
    C. 5 mg po bid
    D. 5 mg po tid

CASE 11

Marcus Green, MD
100 Hospital Drive
Chicago, IL 52111

Patient: Grace Grinder

Date: March 31, 2003

Zonegran 100 mg
30
1 tab po qd

Refill: 3

Doctor: Marcus Green

PHARMACY PROFILE

Patient: Grace Grinder

Patient Weight: 50 kg   **Age:** 7 y/o

Medical History: Partial seizures

Allergies: Lasix

Medication Profile:

Date	Medication	Quantity
01/12/03	Tegretol 400 mg XR bid	60

11a. Which of the following products contains carbamazepine?

   A. Tegretol
   B. Carbatrol
   C. Cerebyx
   D. A and B only
   E. A, B, and C

11b. Which of the following best describes the proposed mechanism of action of Tegretol for the treatment of seizures?

   A. Blockade of sodium channels
   B. Enhances GABA activity
   C. Produces a systemic metabolic acidosis mimicking a ketogenic diet
   D. Reduces voltage-dependent calcium conductance

11c. Despite compliance, Grace's Tegretol serum concentrations declined during the initial 2 weeks of therapy. The most likely explanation would be _____.

   A. decreased bioavailability during adolescence
   B. auto-induction of metabolism
   C. drug-drug interaction
   D. altered protein binding

11d. The active metabolite of carbamazepine is _____.

   A. carbamazepine 10, 11-epoxide
   B. carbamazepine 10-hydroxide
   C. hydroxycarbamazepine
   D. nor-carbamazepine

11e. Which of the following conditions is associated with Tegretol therapy?

  A. Hyponatremic hyperosmolar condition
  B. Hypernatremic hyperosmolar condition
  C. Hypernatremic hyposmolar condition
  D. Hyponatremic hyposmolar condition

11f. The accepted therapeutic serum concentration range for Tegretol is _____ mcg/mL.

  A. 4–12
  B. 10–20
  C. 15–40
  D. 50–100

11g. Which of the following is a keto analogue of carbamazepine?

  A. Trileptal
  B. Sabril
  C. Gabitril
  D. Zarontin

11h. Carbamazepine is available in which of the following dosage forms?

  A. Chewable tablets
  B. Suspension
  C. Extended release capsules
  D. A and B only
  E. A, B, and C

11i. Which of the following anticonvulsants would most likely be associated with an anticonvulsant hypersensitivity syndrome?

  A. Carbamazepine
  B. Phenytoin
  C. Phenobarbital
  D. A and B only
  E. A, B, and C

11j. The active ingredient of Zonegran is _____.

  A. zolmitriptan
  B. zolpidem
  C. ziprasidone
  D. zonisamide

11k. The mechanism of action of Zonegran is believed to be via _____.

  A. potentiation of GABA activity
  B. blockade of sodium and calcium channels
  C. blockade chloride channels
  D. diminishing aspartate activity

11l. Zonegran has proven successful in the treatment of which of the following types of seizures?

  A. Tonic-clonic
  B. Partial
  C. Absence
  D. A and B only
  E. A, B, and C

11m. Which of the following is a side effect associated with Zonegran therapy?

  A. Insomnia
  B. Weight gain
  C. Renal Calculi
  D. Pancreatitis

11n. There is no evidence that exceeding a Zonegran dose of _____ mg/day will result in increased effects.

  A. 100
  B. 200
  C. 300
  D. 400

11o. Zonegran should be used with caution in Grace because _____.

  A. carbamazepine may increase Zonegran serum concentrations
  B. it is not indicated in patients younger than 18 years of age
  C. no therapeutic range has been established
  D. of her Lasix allergy

11p. Zonegran is available in which of the following dosage forms?

  A. Capsules
  B. Tablets
  C. Suspension
  D. A and B only
  E. A, B, and C

CASE 12

Brent Madden, MD
700 Glover Street
Garner, NC 27529

Patient: Victor Clark

Date: April 18, 2003

Tobi 30 mg
60
1 inhalation qid

Refill: 2

Doctor: Brent Madden

PHARMACY PROFILE

Patient: Victor Clark

Patient Weight: 50 kg   **Age:** 17 y/o

Medical History: Cystic fibrosis

Allergies: None

Medication Profile:

Date	Medication	Quantity
03/22/03	ADEK 2 tabs po qd	60
03/22/03	Pancrease MT 10 4 caps w/ meals	120
03/22/03	Pancrease MT 10 1 cap w/ snacks	90

12a. The dose of Pancrease MT is based on which component of the medication?

A. Lipase
B. Amylase
C. Protease
D. Dornase

12b. Which of the following would be an appropriate counseling tip for Victor regarding his Pancrease MT?

A. The capsules should be swallowed whole
B. The capsules may be opened and the contents mixed with a small quantity of applesauce
C. The contents of the capsules may be chewed if followed with a glass of milk
D. A and B only
E. A, B, and C

12c. Which of the following products contains the same active ingredient as Pancrease?

A. Viokase
B. Creon
C. Ultrase
D. A and B only
E. A, B, and C

12d. Victor is prescribed to receive _____ IU of vitamin D per day.

A. 200
B. 400
C. 600
D. 800

12e. The amount of vitamin E in each ADEK tablet is
_____ IU.

A. 75
B. 150
C. 300
D. 600

12f. Which of the following is a component of ADEK tablets?

A. Beta carotene
B. Zinc
C. Folic acid
D. A and B only
E. A, B, and C

12g. Tobi is classified as a(n) _____.

A. penicillin
B. aminoglycoside
C. carbapenem
D. cephalosporin

12h. The active ingredient in Tobi is _____.

A. gentamicin
B. amikacin
C. neomycin
D. tobramycin

12i. Tobi is prescribed to Victor for the treatment of which respiratory pathogen?

A. *Staphylococcus*
B. *Pseudomonas*
C. *Streptococcus*
D. *E. coli*

12j. Which of the following beneficial effects has been reported with the use of Tobi in patients with Cystic fibrosis?

A. Improved pulmonary function
B. Decreased hospitalizations
C. Improved weight gain
D. A and B only
E. A, B, and C

12k. Which of the following represents the targeted serum concentration of the active ingredient in Tobi for Victor?

A. 3–5 mcg/mL
B. 6–8 mcg/mL
C. 8–10 mcg/mL
D. Serum concentrations are not routinely monitored

12l. Tobi is available as a nebulizer solution containing _____.

A. 150 mg/mL
B. 150 mg/5 mL
C. 300 mg/mL
D. 300 mg/5 mL

12m. The correct Tobi regimen for Victor is

_____.

A. 150 mg bid
B. 150 mg tid
C. 300 mg bid
D. 300 mg tid

12n. Which of the following would be an appropriate Tobi cycle for Victor?

A. 7 days on, 7 days off
B. 14 days on, 14 days off
C. 21 days on, 21 days off
D. 28 days on, 28 days off

12o. Which of the following is an adverse effect associated with Tobi therapy?

A. Tinnitus
B. Alteration of voice
C. Nephrotoxicity
D. A and B only
E. A, B, and C

CASE 13

Michael Sneed, MD
300 Rainbow Drive
Cleveland, OH 37689

Patient: Stephen Anderson

Date: May 9, 2003

Dornase alpha
#30
5 mg qid

Refill: 3

Doctor: Michael Sneed

PHARMACY PROFILE

Patient: Stephen Anderson

Patient Weight: 30 kg   **Age:** 10 y/o

Medical History: Cystic fibrosis

Allergies: None

Medication Profile:

Date	Medication	Quantity
04/03/03	ADEK 1 po qd	30
04/03/03	Pancrease MT 4 1 po w/ snacks	90
04/03/03	Pancrease MT 10 1 po w/ meals	90
04/03/03	Motrin 300 mg po q 6 h	120

13a. Ibuprofen is marketed as _____.

   A. Feldene
   B. Clinoril
   C. Orudis
   D. Motrin

13b. Which of the following outcomes has been reported in cystic fibrosis patients treated with ibuprofen?

   A. Improved FEV_1
   B. Better weight maintenance
   C. Less hospital days
   D. A and B only
   E. A, B, and C

13c. Which of the following would tend to occur more frequently in cystic fibrosis patients treated with corticosteroids versus ibuprofen?

   A. Growth retardation
   B. Glucose intolerance
   C. Adrenal suppression
   D. A and B only
   E. A, B, and C

13d. A reasonable targeted ibuprofen serum concentration in Stephen would be _____ mcg/mL.

   A. 10–20
   B. 15–40
   C. 50–100
   D. 100–150

13e. A more appropriate ibuprofen regimen for Stephen would be _____.

 A. 300 mg po bid
 B. 300 mg po tid
 C. 600 mg po bid
 D. 600 mg po tid

13f. How many milliliters of an ibuprofen 100 mg/5 mL suspension would be required to provide Stephen with his daily dose as prescribed?

 A. 20 mL
 B. 40 mL
 C. 60 mL
 D. 80 mL

13g. The brand name for dornase alpha is _____.

 A. Pulmozyme
 B. Pulmicort
 C. Protonix
 D. Protopam

13h. Which of the following is a synonym for dornase alpha?

 A. RNase
 B. DNase
 C. ANase
 D. RDNase

13i. Which of the following best describes the mechanism of action of dornase alpha?

 A. Hydrolyzes DNA in pulmonary secretions
 B. Inhibits neutrophil aggregation
 C. Disrupts replication of gram-negative bacteria
 D. Enhances pancreatic enzyme activity

13j. The correct initial dose of dornase alpha for Stephen is _____.

 A. 2.5 mg daily
 B. 2.5 mg twice daily
 C. 5 mg daily
 D. 5 mg twice daily

13k. Which route of administration is appropriate for dornase alpha?

 A. Oral
 B. Intravenous
 C. Subcutaneous
 D. Inhalation

13l. Which of the following is true regarding dornase alpha?

 A. Should be stored at room temperature
 B. Must be diluted with water prior to use
 C. Potential adverse effects include rash and pharyngitis
 D. A and B only
 E. A, B, and C

CASE 14

Paul Bird, MD
505 Elm Street
St. Louis, MO 28282

Patient: Jack Anderson

Date: April 23, 2003

Hydroxyurea 250 mg
60
1 po bid

Refill: 3

Doctor: Paul Bird

PHARMACY PROFILE

Patient: Jack Anderson

Patient Weight: 50 kg   **Age:** 14 y/o

Medical History: Sickle cell disease

Allergies: None

Medication Profile:

Date	Medication	Quantity
3/25/03	Folic acid	30
3/25/03	Ibuprofen 400 mg po q 6 h prn	100

14a. Sickle cell disease is characterized by the substitution of a _____ for a glutamine at the sixth position of the β-hemoglobin chain.

A. alanine
B. valine
C. tyrosine
D. guanine

14b. A leading cause of death among sickle cell patients is _____ sepsis.

A. *Staphylococcal*
B. *Pseudomonal*
C. *Pneumococcal*
D. *E.coli*

14c. Which of the following conditions promotes polymerization of hemoglobin?

A. Anemia
B. Deoxygenation
C. Leukocytosis
D. Sepsis

14d. Which of the following is a potential vaso-occlusive complication among sickle cell patients?

A. CVA
B. Acute chest syndrome
C. Priapism
D. A and B only
E. A, B, and C

14e. Folic acid is prescribed to Jack to prevent _____.

A. megaloblastic erythropoiesis
B. splenic sequestration
C. pernicious anemia
D. vaso-occlusive events

14f. The correct dose of folic acid for Jack is _____.

A. 1 mcg qd
B. 1 mcg bid
C. 1 mg qd
D. 1 mg bid

14g. Hydroxyurea is classified as a(n) _____.

    A. antibiotic
    B. antineoplastic agent
    C. anticoagulant
    D. colony-stimulating factor

14h. Which of the following is the desired mechanism of action of hydroxyurea for Jack?

    A. Inhibition of thymidine incorporation into DNA
    B. Increased production of fetal hemoglobin
    C. Increased splenic sequestration of sickle hemoglobin
    D. Demargination of red blood cells

14i. Of the following labs, which one deserves preferential monitoring in Jack?

    A. Complete blood count
    B. C-reactive protein
    C. Ammonia
    D. Creatinine

14j. Which of the following counseling tips would be appropriate for Jack regarding his hydroxyurea therapy?

    A. Not all patients respond well to therapy
    B. Ideally, the dose should be taken on an empty stomach
    C. Therapy should not exceed 3 successive months
    D. A and B only
    E. A, B, and C

14k. Of the following lab values, which one would most likely become elevated during hydroxyurea therapy?

    A. Uric Acid
    B. Calcium
    C. Potassium
    D. Sodium

14l. The maximum recommended pediatric daily dose of hydroxyurea is _____ mg/kg/day.

    A. 10
    B. 20
    C. 35
    D. 45

14m. Hydroxyurea is marketed as _____.

    A. Hytone
    B. Hydrea
    C. Hivid
    D. Hytrin

14n. Hydroxyurea is available in which of the following dosage forms?

    A. Tablets
    B. Capsules
    C. Sustained-release tablets
    D. A and B only
    E. A, B, and C

14o. A more appropriate initial regimen of hydroxyurea for Jack is _____.

    A. 250 mg po qd
    B. 500 mg po qd
    C. 500 mg po bid
    D. 750 mg po qd

CASE 15

Larry Smith, MD
300 Carolina Lane
Wilmington, NC 28765

Patient: Beverly Cole

Date: June 22, 2003

Nelfinavir 250 mg
1 month supply
1 po tid

Refill: 3

Doctor: Larry Smith

PHARMACY PROFILE

Patient: Beverly Cole

Medical History: HIV

Medication Profile:

Patient Weight: 25 kg **Age:** 10 y/o

BSA: 0.85 m²

Allergies: None

Date	Medication	Quantity
6/22/03	ddI 100 mg	1 bottle
6/22/03	Zidovudine 150 mg qid	1 bottle

15a. Which of the following is a treatment goal for Beverly?

A. Improved quality of life
B. Suppression of HIV replication
C. Increase in CD4 lymphocytes
D. A and B only
E. A, B, and C

15b. Which of the following is characteristic of children who present with HIV?

A. Obesity
B. Recurrent mild infections
C. Early pubertal development
D. Less severe episodes of childhood illnesses

15c. Which of the following tests was most likely used to diagnose HIV in Beverly?

A. Sputum culture HIV
B. Blood culture for HIV
C. Elisa test for anti-HIV antibodies
D. HIV DNA-polymerase chain reaction (PCR) on peripheral blood lymphocytes

15d. For Beverly, moderate immunosuppression would be defined by a CD4+ T-lymphocyte count between _____.

A. 0–200
B. 200–499
C. 500–999
D. 750–1499

15e. Nelfinavir is marketed as _____.

A. Viracept
B. Norvir
C. Invirase
D. Crixivan

15f. Nelfinavir is classified as a _____.

    A. protease inhibitor
    B. nucleoside reverse transcriptase inhibitor
    C. non-nucleoside reverse transcriptase inhibitor
    D. RNA-polymerase inhibitor

15g. Which of the following medications is most similar to nelfinavir?

    A. Ritonavir
    B. Didanosine
    C. Zidovudine
    D. Lamivudine

15h. Which of the following is true regarding the powder dosage form of nelfinavir?

    A. Is available in a concentration of 100 mg of nelfinavir per gram of powder
    B. Should be reconstituted in the original container
    C. Preferably should be mixed with an acidic beverage
    D. Once mixed, should be used within 6 hours

15i. A more appropriate regimen of nelfinavir for Beverly would have been _____.

    A. 100 mg tid
    B. 300 mg tid
    C. 450 mg tid
    D. 750 mg tid

15j. Didanosine is marketed as _____.

    A. Epivir
    B. Zerit
    C. Hivid
    D. Videx

15k. Didanosine is a synthetic purine nucleoside analogue of _____.

    A. deoxyadenosine
    B. deoxycytidine
    C. thymidine
    D. deoxyguanosine

15l. Which of the following is a severe and potentially fatal adverse effect associated with didanosine?

    A. Pancreatitis
    B. Hepatomegaly
    C. Lactic acidosis
    D. A and B only
    E. A, B, and C

15m. Which of the following is true regarding the ddI pediatric powder for oral solution that was dispensed to Beverly?

    A. The final concentration of a properly prepared solution is 20 mg/mL
    B. Antacids are used to prepare the final dilution
    C. The final reconstituted product is stable for 30 days at room temperature
    D. A and B only
    E. A, B, and C

15n. Beverly's ddI should be taken _____.

    A. once a day
    B. twice a day
    C. three times a day
    D. four times a day

15o. Besides the pediatric oral solution dispensed to Beverly, ddI is also available as a _____.

    A. buffered tablet
    B. buffered powder for oral solution
    C. delayed-release capsule
    D. A and B only
    E. A, B, and C

15p. Zidovudine is also known as _____.

    A. Retrovir
    B. AZT
    C. Azidothymidine
    D. A and B only
    E. A, B, and C

15q. Zidovudine is classified as a _____.

    A. protease inhibitor
    B. nucleoside reverse transcriptase inhibitor
    C. non-nucleoside reverse transcriptase inhibitor
    D. RNA polymerase inhibitor

15r. Which of the following adverse effects is associated with zidovudine therapy?

    A. Lactic acidosis
    B. Granulocytopenia
    C. Myopathy
    D. A and B only
    E. A, B, and C

15s. Zidovudine is available in which of the following dosage forms?

A. Capsules
B. Injection
C. Syrup
D. A and B only
E. A, B, and C

15t. The maximum dose of zidovudine recommended for children < 12 years of age is _____.

A. 100 mg po qid
B. 150 mg po qid
C. 200 mg po qid
D. 250 mg po qid

CASE 16

Laura Boyle, MD
750 Palm Drive
Palm Beach, FL 33708

Patient: Kris Matthews   **Date:** February 20, 2003

Kaletra solution 80 mg/mL
1 month supply
200 mg po bid

Refill: 3   **Doctor:** Laura Boyle

PHARMACY PROFILE

Patient: Kris Matthews   **Patient Weight:** 20 kg   **Age:** 8 y/o

Medical History: HIV   **BSA:** 0.8 m²

Medication Profile: **Allergies:** None

Date	Medication	Quantity
01/18/03	Nelfinavir 500 mg tid	
01/18/03	Stavudine 40 mg tid	90
01/18/03	Lamivudine 150 mg bid	60

16a. To provide Kris with a 30-day supply, she would have been dispensed _____ dosage units of nelfinavir.

   A. 45
   B. 90
   C. 180
   D. 360

16b. Stavudine is also known as _____.

   A. d4T
   B. 3TC
   C. ddI
   D. AZT

16c. Stavudine is marketed as _____.

   A. Zerit
   B. Epivir
   C. Hivid
   D. Videx

16d. Stavudine is classified as a _____.

   A. protease inhibitor
   B. nucleoside-reverse transcriptase inhibitor
   C. non–nucleoside-reverse transcriptase inhibitor
   D. DNA polymer inhibitor

16e. Which of the following is true regarding the peripheral neuropathy associated with stavudine therapy?

   A. Appears to be dose related
   B. Symptoms may worsen temporarily following discontinuation of therapy
   C. Upon resolution, may consider restarting therapy at 75% of the initial dose
   D. A and B only
   E. A, B, and C

16f. The correct regimen of stavudine for Kris would be _____.

A. 20 mg po bid
B. 20 mg po tid
C. 30 mg po bid
D. 30 mg po tid

16g. Lamivudine is also known as _____.

A. d4T
B. ddI
C. AZT
D. 3TC

16h. Which of the following is true regarding the metabolism/elimination of lamivudine?

A. Is predominantly metabolized via the P450 isoenzyme system
B. The P450 3A isoenzyme pathway is the primary route of metabolism
C. Most of the drug is eliminated as unchanged drug in the urine
D. Both A and B

16i. Lamivudine is classified as a _____.

A. protease inhibitor
B. nucleoside-reverse transcriptase inhibitor
C. nonnucleoside-reverse transcriptase inhibitor
D. DNA polymer inhibitor

16j. A more appropriate regimen of lamivudine for Kris is ____ milligrams po bid.

A. 20
B. 40
C. 60
D. 80

16k. Besides HIV, lamivudine is also indicated for the treatment of _____.

A. Crohn's disease
B. Hepatitis B
C. Cytomegalovirus
D. Herpes

16l. Kaletra is a combination product of _____.

A. lopinavir and ritonavir
B. amprenavir and tenovir
C. lopinavir and amprenavir
D. ritonavir and tenovir

16m. Which of the following is true regarding the components of Kaletra?

A. Both components are nucleoside-reverse transcriptase inhibitors
B. Both components are nonnucleoside-reverse transcriptase inhibitors
C. One component inhibits the metabolism of the other
D. One component induces the metabolism of the other

16n. Which of the following is a potential adverse effect from Kaletra therapy?

A. Pancreatitis
B. Diabetes mellitus
C. Hyperlipidemia
D. A and B only
E. A, B, and C

16o. As prescribed, how many milliliters of Kaletra solution should Kris receive per day?

A. 2.5 mL
B. 5 mL
C. 7.5 mL
D. 10 mL

16p. The dose of Kaletra is based on the _____ component of the combination product.

A. ritonavir
B. lopinavir
C. amprenavir
D. tenovir

16q. Which of Kris' medications should be discontinued once Kaletra therapy is initiated?

A. Nelfinavir
B. Stavudine
C. Lamivudine
D. A and B only
E. A, B, and C

CASE 17

Jerry Barone, MD
109 Park Drive
Seattle, WA 56555

Patient: Tricia Stone   **Date:** March 31, 2003

Lantus
1 vial
4 units qd

Refill: 3   **Doctor:** Jerry Barone

PHARMACY PROFILE

Patient: Tricia Stone   **Patient Weight:** 20 kg   **Age:** 6 y/o

Medical History: Type I diabetes   **Allergies:** None

Medication Profile:

Date	Medication	Quantity
02/15/03	Humulin R 3 u q am, 2 u q pm	1 vial
02/15/03	Humulin N 7 u q am, 3 u q pm	1 vial

17a. Which of the following statements is true regarding Type I Diabetes?

    A. Accounts for most of the diabetic population
    B. A strong family history of diabetes is usually present
    C. Patients are prone to ketoacidosis
    D. A and B only
    E. A, B, and C

17b. Which of the following is a potential long-term consequence of poorly controlled diabetes mellitus?

    A. Nephropathy
    B. Blindness
    C. Neuropathy
    D. A and B only
    E. A, B, and C

17c. By definition, a fasting blood glucose concentration greater than _____ mg/dL is diagnostic for diabetes mellitus?

    A. 110
    B. 126
    C. 140
    D. 200

17d. Hemoglobin A_{1c} is an indicator of glucose control over the past _____.

    A. 12–24 hours
    B. 7–14 days
    C. 2–4 weeks
    D. 2–3 months

17e. The absorption of insulin is most rapid from injections in the _____.

    A. abdomen
    B. deltoid
    C. thigh
    D. buttocks

17f. Which of the following is an adverse effect associated with insulin therapy?

A. Hypoglycemia
B. Lipoatrophy
C. Lipohypertrophy
D. A and B only
E. A, B, and C

17g. Which of the following insulin products is the most rapid acting?

A. Humulin N
B. Humulin R
C. Ultralente
D. Humalog

17h. The time required for the onset of the effects from a dose of Humulin R is approximately _____ hours.

A. 0.25
B. 0.5–1.0
C. 1–2
D. 2–4

17i. Which of the following is true regarding Humulin R?

A. May be administered intravenously
B. Is a clear solution
C. Is available as a combination product containing Humulin N 60 units and Humulin R 40 units per milliliter
D. A and B only
E. A, B, and C

17j. The duration of action of Humulin N is approximately _____ hours.

A. 6
B. 12
C. 18
D. 24

17k. Which of the following counseling tips should Tricia have received regarding the withdrawal of both her Humulin insulins in the same syringe prior to injecting?

A. Withdraw the Humulin R first, followed by the Humulin N
B. Withdraw the Humulin N first, followed by the Humulin R
C. The order in which they are withdrawn is of no consequence
D. Do not mix the insulins in the same syringe

17l. How many milliliters of Humulin N should Tricia receive for her prescribed morning dose?

A. 0.07 mL
B. 0.7 mL
C. 7 mL
D. 70 mL

17m. Lantus is also known as _____.

A. insulin glargine
B. insulin lispro
C. isophane insulin
D. insulin protamine

17n. Which of the following routes of administration is appropriate for Lantus?

A. Intravenous
B. Subcutaneous
C. Intramuscular
D. A and B only
E. A, B, and C

17o. Which of the following is true regarding Lantus?

A. It should be diluted prior to use
B. It may be mixed in the same syringe with short-acting insulins
C. Its constant glucose-lowering action allows for once daily dosing
D. A and B only
E. A, B, and C

17p. As prescribed, Tricia should receive her Lantus dose _____.

A. in the morning
B. at noon
C. at bedtime
D. whenever desired as long as the time is consistent from day to day.

17q. A more appropriate initial Lantus dose for Tricia would be _____.

A. 4 units bid
B. 8 units qd
C. 10 units qd
D. 12 units qd

CASE 18

Elizabeth Barber, MD
100 Professional Lane
Chicago, IL 23345

Patient: Martha Miller

Date: August 19, 2003

Metformin tabs
60
1 po bid

Refill: 3

Doctor: Elizabeth Barber

PHARMACY PROFILE

Patient: Martha Miller

Patient Weight: 50 kg   **Age:** 12 y/o

Medical History: Diabetes mellitus

Allergies: None

Medication Profile:

Date	Medication	Quantity
06/19/03	Septra DS 1 po bid	20

18a. Which of the following is true of children diagnosed with Type II diabetes?

A. Most of the children are overweight or obese
B. A family history of diabetes is usually present
C. Most patients present with severe polyuria and weight loss
D. A and B only
E. A, B, and C

18b. Which of the following is an acceptable criteria for screening children for Type II Diabetes?

A. Overweight plus additional risks factors including race and family history
B. Begin screening at age 16 years or at onset of puberty
C. Oral Glucose Tolerance Test and HbA_{1c} are the preferred screening labs
D. A and B only
E. A, B, and C

18c. Which of the following is a goal in the treatment of children with Type II diabetes?

A. Normalization of blood-glucose concentrations
B. Decrease microvascular complications
C. Control associated comorbidities such as hypertension and hyperlipidemia
D. A and B only
E. A, B, and C

18d. Which of the following is true of lifestyle changes in children with Type II diabetes?

A. Lifestyle changes should include diet and exercise
B. Lifestyle changes can result in successful diabetes management in ~ 25% of patients.
C. Successful lifestyle changes would be defined by a fasting blood-glucose concentration between 140–160 mg/dL
D. A and B only
E. A, B, and C

18e. Metformin is marketed as _____.

A. Avandia
B. Glucophage
C. Precose
D. Actos

18f. Metformin is classified as a _____.

A. biguanide
B. sulfonylurea
C. meglitinide
D. glucosidase inhibitor

18g. Which of the following is associated with metformin therapy?

A. Decrease in LDL cholesterol concentrations
B. Decrease in triglyceride concentrations
C. Risk of hypoglycemia
D. A and B only
E. A, B, and C

18h. Which of the following is a rare, but serious complication of metformin therapy?

A. Lactic acidosis
B. Pancreatitis
C. Renal failure
D. Hepatitis

18i. Martha should be prescribed _____ milligram tablets for her metformin prescription.

A. 250
B. 500
C. 850
D. 1000

18j. Besides the one prescribed to Martha, metformin is also available in which of the following dosage forms?

A. Extended-release tablet
B. Oral solution
C. Capsule
D. A and B only
E. A, B, and C

MODULE 4 ANSWERS

CASE 1

1a. (B) Acute otitis media is defined by middle ear fluid in the presence of signs and symptoms of infection. Otitis media with effusion refers to middle ear fluid in the absence of local or systemic illness.

1b. (D) Acute otitis media typically follows a viral infection and is the most common reason for prescribing medications to children. It occurs more commonly in males.

1c. (E) Other risk factors include immature immune systems, presence of siblings with recurrent otitis media, winter season, Caucasian race, crowded living conditions, poor sanitary conditions, and congenital malformations.

1d. (C)

1e. (D) Augmentin consists of an antibiotic, amoxicillin, and a β-lactamase inhibitor, potassium clavulanate.

1f. (B) Like sulbactam and potassium clavulanate, tazobactam is also a β-lactamase inhibitor. β-lactamase inhibitors prevent the bacteria's β-lactamase from disrupting the antibiotic's β-lactam ring thus rendering the antibiotic effective in eradicating the β-lactamase producing bacteria.

1g. (B) The potassium clavulanate component of Augmentin is often implicated in causing diarrhea.

1h. (C) Beverly was prescribed 125 mg three times a day or 375 mg per day. Using a 125 mg/5 mL suspension, she would require 15 mL per day; 125 mg/5 mL = 375 mg/x; x = 15 mL. Therefore, 15 mL/day = 150 mL/x; x = 10 days.

1i. (C) Augmentin may be taken with or without food. Both the 250- and 500-mg tablets contain the same quantity of potassium clavulanate (125 mg), so they cannot be interchanged. The dose of Augmentin is based on the antibiotic component (amoxicillin) of the product.

1j. (A)

1k. (B) Beverly is prescribed 1 teaspoonful or ~ 5 mL of Amoxil three times a day for 7 days. Therefore, 5 mL × 3 times a day × 7 days = 105 mL or ~ 100 mLs.

1l. (D) Since Amoxil is a suspension, it should be shaken well before use. Beverly should be treated for the entire course prescribed with any remaining drug discarded at that time. Terminating treatment early may result in treatment failure and/or the emergence of resistant bacteria.

1m. (C) For the treatment of otitis media, a newly established dosing regimen for amoxicillin is 80–90 mg/kg/day divided into two doses. Therefore, Beverly should receive 450 mg po twice a day (10 kg × 90 mg/kg/day divided two times daily = 450 mg twice a day).

1n. (D) The reasoning for the recommended increased dose of amoxicillin is a result of the increasing prevalence of resistant *Streptococcal pneumoniae*.

1o. (D) Although not considered the drugs of choice for otitis media, both Zithromax and Rocephin may be administered as single doses of 30 mg/kg and 50 mg/kg, respectively.

CASE 2

2a. (B) Ventolin and Proventil are brand name products of albuterol.

2b. (D) Albuterol (Ventolin) is a β-2 agonist that acts as a quick-acting bronchodilator in asthma patients. It is considered a rescue medication for these patients.

2c. (C) Each actuation of a Ventolin metered dose inhaler delivers 90 mcg of albuterol.

2d. (E) Inhaled albuterol is usually well tolerated by most patients. The most common complaints include nervousness, tachycardia, and restlessness. Although not usually clinically significant, albuterol can cause an intracellular shift of potassium yielding a reduced serum-potassium concentration.

2e. (E) Ventolin is available in several dosage forms including tablets, oral syrup, metered dose inhaler, solution for inhalation, and capsules for inhalation.

2f. (D) Vanceril Double Strength inhaler provides 84 mcg of beclomethasone dipropionate per activation.

2g. (A) Vanceril (beclomethasone) is classified as an inhaled corticosteroid.

2h. (D) Vanceril Double Strength inhaler provides 84 mcg of beclomethasone dipropionate per actuation (puff). Since Todd is prescribed 2 puffs, he will receive 168 mcg per dose (2 × 84 mcg = 168 mcg).

2i. (C) Inhaled corticosteroids such as Vanceril are usually devoid of systemic side effects. The most common adverse effects include hoarseness and oral thrush which may be prevented by rinsing the mouth well after dosing or using a spacer. However, systemic adverse effects may manifest with the use of high dose inhaled corticosteroids.

2j. (C) Aerobid contains the active ingredient flunisolide. Like beclomethasone, it is also an inhaled corticosteroid.

2k. (C) In the event an inhaled corticosteroid and rapid-acting β-agonist are dosed at the same time, the β-agonist should be dosed first. The rapid-acting β-agonist will cause acute bronchodilation allowing for more of the corticosteroid dose to be delivered to the airways. Therefore, in this case, the Ventolin (β-agonist) should be dosed first.

2l. (B) Advair contains a corticosteroid (fluticasone propionate) and a long-acting β-2 agonist (salmeterol).

2m. (C) Advair is only available in a Diskus device in three dosages. Each of the three dosages contain the same quantity of salmeterol (50 mcg) combined with either 100, 250, or 500 mcg of fluticasone. Since Advair doesn't contain an immediate-acting β-2 agonists, it is not indicated for the treatment of acute asthma exacerbations.

2n. (A) Since Advair is not indicated for acute asthma exacerbations, prescribing a rapid-acting β-2 agonist, such as albuterol, to dose for acute asthma exacerbations would be appropriate.

2o. (B)

CASE 3

3a. (B) Xopenex contains the active R-enantiomer of albuterol, levalbuterol.

3b. (B)

3c. (D) The recommended dose of Xopenex is 0.63 or 1.25 mg three times a day, every 6–8 hours.

3d. (B) Xopenex is only available as a solution for inhalation via nebulization.

3e. (B)

3f. (B)

3g. (C) Singulair is extensively metabolized via the liver and does not necessitate dosage adjustments in the presence of renal dysfunction. It is available in 4- and 5-mg chewable tablets and a 10-mg tablet.

3h. (E) Zafirlukast (Accolate) and zileuton (Zyflo) are also leukotriene antagonists. While Singulair is

dosed once daily, Accolate and Zyflo are dosed two and four times a day, respectively. Zyflo is a known hepatotoxin and is contraindicated with active liver disease or when transaminase concentrations are greater than 3 times the upper limit. Unlike Accolate and Zyflo, Singulair has a pediatric indication.

3i. (C) The adult dose of Singulair is 10 mg po qd. For children 6–14 years of age, a daily dose of 5 mg is recommended. A daily dose of 4 mg is indicated for children 2–5 years of age.

3j. (D) Flovent contains the active ingredient fluticasone propionate.

3k. (B)

3l. (D) Tracy is prescribed albuterol 2.5 mg or 0.0025 gms. The solution prescribed is 0.083% or 0.083 gm/100 mL. Therefore, 0.083 gms/100 mL = 0.0025 gms/x; x = 3 mLs.

3m. (D) Based on the available literature, Xopenex (levalbuterol) is no more effective or safe than racemic albuterol. As a result of the increased cost of Xopenex, albuterol remains the β-2 agonist drug of choice for acute exacerbations of asthma.

3n. (D) Using reliever medications, such as albuterol, indicates poor control of asthma and the possibility of worsening asthma. In such cases, controller medications should be reassessed with the medication regimen adjusted to attain better control.

CASE 4

4a. (A) The total prescribed dose is 300 mg (100 mg on day 1, then 50 mg a day for 4 days = 300 mg); Therefore, 100 mg/5 mL = 300 mg/x; x = 15 mL.

4b. (D) Alternative azithromycin regimens for otitis media are 30 mg/kg as a single dose or 10 mg/kg once daily for 3 days. Therefore, for Gary, 300 mg (30 mg/kg × 10 kg) once or 100 mg (10 mg/kg × 10 kg) qd for 3 days.

4c. (B) A single dose of ceftriaxone (Rocephin) 50 mg/kg IM may be used as an alternative therapy for the treatment of otitis media. For resistant bacteria, a 3-day regimen of 50 mg/kg/day is recommended.

4d. (B) IPV means "inactivated polio vaccine." It consists of three types of poliovirus grown in monkey kidney cells and inactivated with formaldehyde.

4e. (C) Children should receive four doses of IPV at ages 2 months, 4 months, 6–18 months, and 4–6 years. Therefore, Gary should have received two doses prior to his dose at 12 months of age.

4f. (B) The second dose of MMR is usually given at age 4–6 years, but may be given at any time provided at least 4 weeks have elapsed since the first dose and that both doses are given beginning at or after 12 months of age.

4g. (A) Measles, mumps, and rubella is a live, attenuated trivalent vaccine. Two doses are recommended for children. Contrary to recent claims, studies have not confirmed an association between the measles vaccine and an increase in autism.

4h. (A)

4i. (A) When MMR and Varicella vaccines are given fewer than 30 days apart, but not simultaneously, there is an increased incidence of breakthrough varicella.

4j. (B) The respective generic and trade names are valganciclovir (Valcyte), varicella virus vaccine (Varivax), valacyclovir (Valtrex), and ribavirin (Virazole).

4k. (B) For patients older than 13 years of age, two doses of varicella vaccine separated by at least 4 weeks are recommended. Because of the potential risk of Reye's Syndrome, recipients should avoid the use of salicylates for 6 weeks after receiving the varicella vaccine. Although IM administration has resulted in successful seroconversion, the SC route is recommended.

4l. (C) Four doses of pneumococcal vaccine at 2, 4, 6, and 12–15 months are recommended. Therefore, Gary should have received three doses prior to his dose at 12 months of age.

4m. (C) Prevnar is a heptavalent pneumococcal conjugate vaccine recommended for all children ages 2–23 months. Pneumovax 23 and Pnu-Imune 23 are polyvalent pneumococcal vaccines given to adults and children older than 2 years of age.

4n. (B)

4o. (B) Prevnar is the heptavalent pneumococcal vaccine recommended for all children. It is dosed at ages 2, 4, 6, and 12–15 months of age. Since it is not a live vaccine, it can be safely administered to immunocompromised children.

4p. (D) IPV, varicella, and MMR vaccines contain neomycin.

CASE 5

5a. (E) Flura-Drops and Luride drops contain 0.25 and 0.125 mg of fluoride ion per drop, respectively.

Gel Kam is stannous fluoride containing 0.1% fluoride ion.

5b. (A) The appropriate dose of fluoride ion for a patient 6 months to 3 years old with a drinking water fluoride concentration<0.3 ppm is 0.25 mg. Therefore, since Bonnie was prescribed a preparation containing 0.25 mg/drop, she should be given 1 drop or 0.25 mg per day.

5c. (A) All infants should receive the first dose of hepatitis B vaccine soon after birth. The second dose should be given at least 4 weeks after the first dose with the final dose given at least 16 weeks after the first dose, but not before 8 weeks after the second dose and not before 6 months of age.

5d. (C) Neurologic complications including fever, seizures, encephalopathy, and inconsolable crying are associated with the pertussis vaccine. In contrast to whole cell pertussis, the acellular pertussis vaccine is highly effective and appears to result in fewer adverse effects.

5e. (E) Other contraindications to the DTaP vaccine include an anaphylactic reaction to a previous dose, persistent, severe, inconsolable crying or screaming for 3 or more hours within 48 hours of a dose, or a temperature ≥ 40.5 degrees Celsius within 48 hours of a dose.

5f. (A)

5g. (D) Acellular pertussis is now recommended for all five doses of the diphtheria, tetanus, and pertussis vaccine. Doses are given at 2, 4, 6, and 12–18 months and 4–6 years of age.

5h. (B)

5i. (D) Four doses of *Haemophilus influenzae* type-b conjugate vaccine, given at 2, 4, 6, and 12–15 months of age, are recommended.

5j. (D) If the capsular polysaccharide outer membrane protein products of Hib, PedvaxHIB or Comvax, are used, the dose at 6 months of age is not required.

5k. (E) Other Hib products include ActHib and PedvaxHib.

5l. (B) A total of three doses are recommended to complete the hepatitis B vaccine schedule.

5m. (D) Havrix is the trade name for hepatitis A vaccine.

5n. (B) Infants born to HbsAg-positive mothers should receive hepatitis B vaccine and 0.5 mL of hepatitis B immune globulin within 12 hours of birth.

5o. (E) Severely immunosuppressed patients should not receive live vaccines (i.e., MMR and Varicella) owing to a decreased antibody response and potential for serious complications. However, HIV infected infants with adequate CD4 lymphocyte counts (i.e., ≥ 25% total lymphocytes) may receive live vaccines. Such patients should receive the first dose of MMR at 12 months of age with the second dose given as soon as 28 days after the first dose.

CASE 6

6a. (B) Sarah is prescribed 0.25 mL twice a day or 0.5 mL per day. Therefore, she will require 15 mL for a 30 day supply (0.5 mL/day × 30 days = 15 mL).

6b. (D) Sarah is prescribed 0.25 mL twice a day or 0.5 mL per day. The concentration of her Lasix solution is 10 mg/mL. Therefore, 10 mg/1 mL = x/0.5 mL; x = 5 mg.

6c. (A) Palivizumab is a humanized monoclonal antibody produced by recombinant DNA technology. It is indicated for the prevention of lower respiratory tract disease caused by respiratory syncytial virus (RSV). Palivizumab may be given without regard to immunizations.

6d. (B) The respective generic and trade names are quinupristin/dalfopristin (Synercid), palivizumab (Synagis), fluocinolone (Synalar), and hydrocortisone (Synacort).

6e. (B) Palivizumab should be dosed monthly throughout the RSV season. Therefore, Sarah should receive her next dose on December 1, approximately 1 month after her previous dose.

6f. (A) The dose of palivizumab is 15 mg/kg once a month. Therefore, the dose for Sarah is 15 mg/kg × 5 kg = 75 mg.

6g. (C) Palivizumab is administered intramuscularly, preferably in the anterolateral aspect of the thigh. Injection volumes greater than 1 mL should be given in divided doses.

6h. (B) The respective generic and trade names are ribavirin (Virazole), RSV-IVIG (Respigam), palivizumab (Synagis), and immune globulin intravenous (Gamimune N).

6i. (D) The dose of RSV-IVIG is 750 mg/kg once a month. Therefore, the dose for Sarah is 750 mg/kg × 5 kg = 3750 mg. The dose should be administered as follows: 0–15 minutes, 1.5 mL/kg/hr; 15–30 minutes, 3 mL/kg/hr; 30 minutes to end of infusion, 6 mL/kg/hr.

6j. (C) Because of a diminished immunologic response, live vaccines, MMR and varicella, should not be administered with RSV-IVIG. If given within 10 months of RSV-IVIG, re-immunization is recommended. It is given as an intravenous infusion and the vial should not be shaken. Although purification methods are used in the preparation of RSV-IVIG, there exists a potential for the transmission of blood-borne pathogens.

6k. (A) The infusion of RSV-IVIG should begin within 6 hours and is to be completed within 12 hours after entry into the vial.

CASE 7

7a. (E)

7b. (D) Although the mechanism of action of psychostimulants for the treatment of attention deficit hyperactivity disorder is unclear, it is believed to involve the blockade of dopamine and norepinephrine reuptake.

7c. (A)

7d. (A) As typical of psychostimulants, side effects of Ritalin include headache, abdominal pain, anorexia, insomnia, and irritability.

7e. (A) Ritalin is often initiated with a dose in the morning and at noon. If an additional dose is needed, it should be given in the afternoon so as not to interfere with the child's nighttime sleep.

7f. (C)

7g. (B) Concerta is an extended-release formulation of methylphenidate. Its formulation uses an osmotic controlled-release system (OROS) that contains an immediate-release component followed by an extended-release component.

7h. (A) For patients taking Ritalin 5 mg two or three times a day or Ritalin SR 20 mg daily, the initial dose of Concerta should be 18 mg daily. Therefore, since Peter was receiving Ritalin 5 mg three times a day, he should be started on Concerta 18 mg once a day.

7i. (C)

7j. (E) Other contraindications to Concerta therapy include marked tension, agitation, hypersensitivity to the drug, or patients taking monoamine oxidase inhibitors.

CASE 8

8a. (E) The fourth component of Adderall is d,l-amphetamine sulfate.

8b. (B) For patients taking Adderall, the same number of milligrams may be converted to Adderall XR and give once daily. Since Robert is prescribed Adderall 5 mg bid, an initial dose of Adderall XR 10 mg qd would be appropriate.

8c. (B)

8d. (A) Dexmethylphenidate (Focalin) is the d-threo-enantiomer of racemic methylphenidate and is believed to be the active component of the racemic mixture.

8e. (A) The usual starting dose of Focalin for patients not receiving methylphenidate is 2.5 mg twice daily titrated weekly to a maximum dose of 10 mg twice daily. For patients receiving methylphenidate, the initial dose should be one-half the dose of the patient's racemic methylphenidate dose.

8f. (B) The duration of action of Concerta is ~ 12 hours. The duration of action of Ritalin LA, Metadate ER, and Focalin is ~ 8–10 hours, 6–8 hours, and 4–5 hours, respectively.

8g. (C) Cylert (pemoline) is a stimulant medication used in the treatment of ADHD. Because of its associated liver toxicity, Cylert is rarely prescribed and is suggested to only be used in patients failing first and second line therapies.

8h. (D) Although not usually considered first line therapy for ADHD, antidepressants may be beneficial to patients refractory to stimulants or those with coexisting depression.

8i. (B) Tricyclic antidepressants, such as imipramine, are associated with adverse effects including sedation, hypotension (orthostatic), arrhythmias, seizures, and anticholinergic effects (urinary retention, blurred vision, dry mouth, and constipation).

8j. (A) The respective generic and trade names are imipramine (Tofranil), amitriptyline (Elavil), desipramine (Norpramin), and doxepin (Sinequan).

8k. (D) Bupropion (Wellbutrin) is an antidepressant medication. While bupropion therapy does not possess the cardiovascular risks associated with the tricyclic antidepressants, it may elicit seizure activity in predisposed patients such as those with a history of seizures, those with eating disorders, or patients receiving high doses.

8l. (A) Atomoxetine (Strattera) is a nonstimulant medication used in the treatment of ADHD that is believed to act through blockade of the presynaptic norepinephrine transporter in the brain resulting in inhibition of norepinephrine reuptake.

CASE 9

9a. (E) Other examples of generalized seizures include clonic, tonic, atonic, and infantile spasms.

9b. (D) Acetylcholine, norepinephrine, histamine, corticotropin-releasing factor, glutamate, and aspartate are excitatory compounds that can affect neuronal firing and thus elicit seizure activity.

9c. (A) Dilantin injection and capsules contain phenytoin sodium that contains 92% phenytoin. The oral tablets and suspension contain 100% phenytoin.

9d. (A) The mechanism of action of phenytoin (Dilantin) involves inducing voltage and use-dependent blockade of sodium channels.

9e. (B) The accepted therapeutic serum concentration range for phenytoin is 10–20 mcg/mL.

9f. (E) Other potential adverse effects of phenytoin include sedation, tremor, nystagmus, hirsutism, decreased folic acid, peripheral neuropathy, hepatotoxicity, blood dyscrasias, osteoporosis, and inhibition of insulin release.

9g. (B) The recommended initial pediatric Dilantin dose is 5 mg/kg/day divided in 2 or 3 doses with a normal maintenance dose being 5–10 mg/kg/day. Therefore, for Samantha, 50 mg po tid or 150 mg/day is reasonable (5 mg/kg/day × 30 kg = 150 mg/day). Subsequent dosing adjustments should be based on clinical response, adverse effects, and serum concentrations.

9h. (B)

9i. (E)

9j. (D) Topamax is available in both tablet and sprinkle capsule dosage forms. The sprinkle capsules may be swallowed whole or the contents may be sprinkled on a small amount of soft food. The drug/food mixture should be consumed immediately and not chewed.

9k. (D) Other side effects associated with Topamax include mental slowing, fatigue, somnolence, weight loss, dizziness, ataxia, diplopia, nervousness, increased insulin effect, acute myopia, and secondary angle closure glaucoma.

9l. (B) The initial recommended pediatric dose of Topamax is 1 mg/kg/day in two divided doses. The maintenance dose is typically 6–9 mg/kg/day. Therefore, for Samantha, an initial dose of 1 mg/kg/day or 15 mg (1 mg/kg/day × 30 kg = 30 mg/day) po bid is appropriate.

9m. (D) When given concurrently, Topamax may increase Dilantin serum concentrations and Dilantin may decrease Topamax serum concentrations. Concurrent administration of carbamazepine or valproic acid with Topamax may also result in decreased Topamax serum concentrations.

CASE 10

10a. (C)

10b. (E) Valproic acid is also effective for the treatment of myoclonic and absence seizures.

10c. (E) Other potential adverse effects of valproic acid include sedation, alopecia, dementia, hepatotoxicity, thrombocytopenia, tremor, and edema.

10d. (D) Valproic acid therapy may result in hepatotoxicity, therefore occasional liver function tests are warranted, especially during the first 6 months of therapy. Ammonia concentrations may also become elevated during therapy.

10e. (D) Valproic acid serum concentrations up to 150 mcg/mL have been targeted in some patients with refractory seizures.

10f. (C)

10g. (C) The pediatric oral dose of carnitine is 50–100 mg/kg/day in 2–3 divided doses. Therefore, 500 mg po tid would be an appropriate dose for Faith (500 mg × 3 doses/day = 1500 mg/day; 1500 mg/day divided by 25 kg = 60 mg/kg/day).

10h. (A) Lamictal (lamotrigine) is available as oral tablets and oral chewable tablets.

10i. (B) Serious rashes necessitating discontinuation of therapy and hospitalization have occurred during Lamictal therapy. The incidence of rash appears to be higher in pediatric than in adult patients. To decrease the incidence of a rash, it is recommended to begin therapy conservatively and increase the dose slowly as indicated.

10j. (B) In the presence of valproic acid, a P450 isoenzyme inhibitor, Lamictal should be initiated at a dose of ~ 0.15 mg/kg/day in 1 or 2 divided doses for the first 2 weeks of therapy (normal initial dose = 0.5 mg/kg/day). Therefore, for Faith, 0.15 mg/kg/day × 25 kg = 3.75 mg/day or ~ 2 mg po bid.

CASE 11

11a. (D) Tegretol, Tegretol XR (extended release tablets), and Carbatrol (extended release capsules) contain carbamazepine.

11b. (A) The proposed mechanism of action of carbamazepine is prevention of repetitive firing of action potentials in depolarized neurons through voltage and use-dependent blockade of sodium channels.

11c. (B) Not only is carbamazepine an inducer of the cytochrome P450 isoenzyme system, but it also induces its own metabolism. Autoinduction usually dissipates after 2 to 4 weeks of therapy.

11d. (A)

11e. (D) Carbamazepine therapy may result in increased antidiuretic hormone secretion resulting in a hyponatremic hyposmolar condition similar to that seen with SIADH.

11f. (A)

11g. (A)

11h. (E) Carbamazepine is also available in extended-release tablets (Tegretol XR).

11i. (E) The aromatic anticonvulsants (phenytoin, phenobarbital, and carbamazepine) are metabolized partially by the cytochrome P450 isoenzyme system to reactive aromatic epoxide intermediates (arene oxides) that are believed to be responsible for immunologic reactions. Such reactions manifest as a fever, rash, lymphadenopathy, hepatitis, nephritis, and hematologic abnormalities.

11j. (D)

11k. (B) Although the mechanism of action of Zonegran is unknown, it is believed to be via blockade of sodium and calcium channels. It also appears to have weak carbonic anhydrase inhibiting activity.

11l. (E) Zonegran is indicated as adjunctive therapy for the treatment of partial seizures in patients older than 16 years of age. It has also been effective in the treatment of tonic-clonic, absence, atonic, and myoclonic seizures.

11m. (C) Zonegran therapy may result in kidney stone formation. Therefore, adequate fluid intake is recommended during therapy.

11n. (D) Although doses of 600 mg/day of Zonegran have been used, it appears doses in excess of 400 mg/day offer no additional benefit.

11o. (D) Grace's allergy to Lasix may be the result of the sulfur component of Lasix. Therefore, the administration of Zonegran, a sulfonamide, may result in an allergic reaction in Grace.

11p. (A) Zonegran is only available in 100-mg capsules.

CASE 12

12a. (A)

12b. (D) To protect the enteric coating, Pancrease MT should not be crushed or chewed. If patients are unable to swallow the capsule, the contents may be sprinkled on soft food that does not require chewing. The dose should be taken immediately after mixing with food.

12c. (E) Each of these four products contains pancrelipase.

12d. (D) Each tablet of ADEK contains 400 IU of vitamin D. Therefore, Victor will receive 800 IU/day from 2 tablets.

12e. (B)

12f. (E) ADEK tablets also contain vitamins A, D, E, K, C, B1, B2, B6, and B12 and niacin, biotin, and pantothenic acid.

12g. (B)

12h. (D)

12i. (B) Tobi is prescribed for the treatment of *Pseudomonas aeruginosa*, the major gram-negative pulmonary infectious burden in cystic fibrosis patients.

12j. (E) Tobi therapy has also been found to reduce the density of *Pseudomonas* in the sputum of cystic fibrosis patients.

12k. (D) Inhaled Tobi typically does not result in significant serum tobramycin concentrations, and therefore concentrations are not routinely monitored.

12l. (D)

12m. (C) Although various doses of inhaled tobramycin have been used, 300 mg twice a day seems to be the preferred regimen.

12n. (D) The recommended dosing cycle for Tobi is 28 days on therapy followed by 28 days off therapy.

12o. (D) Inhaled tobramycin is considered less toxic than systemically administered tobramycin. The most common adverse effects have been tinnitus and an alteration of voice.

CASE 13

13a. (D) Advil and Motrin-IB are brands of ibuprofen available over the counter. The over the counter strength is 200 mg per dosage unit.

13b. (D) High dose ibuprofen therapy in cystic fibrosis patients has resulted in improved pulmonary function and better maintenance of ideal body weight. However, no significance difference in hospital admissions or number of hospital days has been appreciated.

13c. (E) Corticosteroids have been used to slow the progression of lung disease in cystic fibrosis patients. However, adverse effects including growth retardation and glucose intolerance have resulted in termination of therapy. Adrenal suppression would also be a concern with corticosteroid use.

13d. (C) Studies involving cystic fibrosis patients have targeted ibuprofen concentrations between 50–100 mcg/mL as neutrophils appear to be inhibited at concentrations in excess of 50 mcg/mL.

13e. (C) Ibuprofen doses between 16–32 mg/kg twice a day have been shown to result in serum concentrations between 50–100 mcg/mL in cystic fibrosis patients. For Stephen, 600 mg twice a day would provide him with 20 mg/kg/dose (600 mg/30 kg = 20 mg/kg).

13f. (C) Ibuprofen is available as a 100 mg/5 mL suspension. Stephen is prescribed 1200 mg of ibuprofen daily (300 mg × 4 doses/day = 1200 mg). Therefore, 100 mg/5 mL = 1200 mg/x; x = 60 mL).

13g. (A) The respective generic and trade names are dornase alpha (Pulmozyme), budesonide (Pulmicort), pantoprazole (Protonix), and pralidoxime chloride (Protopam).

13h. (B) Dornase alpha is known as DNase and recombinant human deoxyribonuclease.

13i. (A) Dornase alpha hydrolyzes DNA in pulmonary secretions resulting in less viscous respiratory secretions.

13j. (A) Dornase alpha is typically initially dosed at 2.5 mg once daily with the dose in some patients being increased to twice daily.

13k. (D) Dornase alpha is inhaled via nebulization.

13l. (C) Dornase alpha must be stored in the refrigerator and should not be diluted or mixed with other drugs in the nebulizer.

CASE 14

14a. (B)

14b. (C) Pneumococcal sepsis a major cause of death among sickle cell patients because of damaged spleens not being able to clear pneumococci from the blood.

14c. (B) In sickle cell patients, the mutated hemoglobin polymerizes when deoxygenated resulting in abnormal erythrocyte shape and tendency to occlude the microvasculature.

14d. (E) Other vaso-occlusive complications among sickle cell patients include painful episodes, liver disease, splenic sequestration, abortion, leg ulcers, osteonecrosis, retinopathy, and renal dysfunction.

14e. (A)

14f. (C)

14g. (B) Hydroxyurea is an antineoplastic agent indicated for the treatment of melanoma, chronic myelocytic leukemia, ovarian carcinoma, and as an adjunct to irradiation in the treatment of primary squamous cell carcinomas of the head and neck.

14h. (B) Hydroxyurea increases the production of fetal hemoglobin (Hemoglobin F). In sickle cell patients, hemoglobin F concentrations greater than 20% seem to provide protection against most vaso-occlusive events.

14i. (A) Hydroxyurea therapy is myelosuppressive and therefore necessitates monitoring complete blood counts. Initially, blood counts should be monitored every 2 weeks until a stable dose is achieved. Thereafter, blood counts should be monitored every 4–6 weeks.

14j. (D) Response to hydroxyurea therapy differs among patients. Patients should be told that many months may be required to find the appropriate dose and that strict compliance and frequent laboratory monitoring will be necessary. It should be taken on an empty stomach with water. If unable to swallow, the contents of the capsule may be dissolved in a glass of water and consumed immediately.

14k. (A) Uric acid, blood urea nitrogen, and creatinine concentrations may become elevated during hydroxyurea therapy.

14l. (C) The maintenance dose of hydroxyurea for most pediatric patients with sickle cell disease is 1000–2000 mg per day or 20–30 mg/kg/day. The maximum recommended dose is 35 mg/kg/day or 2500 mg/day.

14m. (B) The respective generic and trade names are hydrocortisone (Hytone), hydroxyurea (Hydrea), zalcitabine (Hivid) and terazosin (Hytrin).

14n. (B) Hydroxyurea is only available in a capsule dosage form.

14o. (B) Hydroxyurea therapy for sickle cell disease is initiated at 500 mg or 10 mg/kg/day. Either way, Jack should be started on 500 mg/day (50 kg × 10 mg/kg/day = 500 mg/day). After 6–8 weeks, the dose may be increased to 1000 mg/day provided blood counts are stable.

CASE 15

15a. (E) The ultimate goal in the treatment of HIV patients is to decrease morbidity and mortality. In doing so, achieving maximal suppression of HIV replication, increasing CD4 lymphocytes, and improving overall quality of life are desirable.

15b. (B) Many children with HIV have only mild symptoms for years. Older children may present with recurrent mild infections or one or more episodes of more severe infections. In such children, common illnesses such as chicken pox may have a longer recovery period. Infections may also be associated with hepatosplenomegaly, lymphadenopathy, or problems of growth and weight gain.

15c. (C) As in adults, in pediatric patients older than 18 months of age, HIV is diagnosed by detection of anti-HIV antibodies in the blood (Elisa-based antibody test). In patients up to 18 months of age, anti-HIV antibody in the serum may be of transplacental origin and not diagnostic of HIV. Therefore, the gold standard test in these patients to detect HIV is the HIV DNA-polymerase chain reaction (PCR) on peripheral blood lymphocytes.

15d. (B) The CD4+ T-lymphocyte counts indicative of moderate suppression are 750–1499, 500–999, and 200–499 cells/μl for patients < 12 months, 1–5 years, and 6–12 years, respectively. The cell counts indicative of severe suppression are < 750, < 500, and < 200 cells/μl, respectively.

15e. (A) The respective generic and trade names are nelfinavir (Viracept), ritonavir (Norvir), saquinavir (Invirase), and indinavir (Crixivan).

15f. (A)

15g. (A) Ritonavir is also a protease inhibitor. Didanosine, zidovudine, and lamivudine are nucleoside reverse transcriptase inhibitors.

15h. (D) Nelfinavir is available as a 50 mg/g powder formulation. It should be mixed with a small amount of water, milk, or soy formula or milk. Acidic products should not be used as diluents because of a resultant bitter taste. Once mixed, it should be given within 6 hours.

15i. (D) The pediatric dose of nelfinavir is 20–30 mg/kg three times a day. Therefore, a reasonable dose for Beverly is 30 mg/kg $\times$ 25 kg = 750 mg three times a day.

15j. (D) The respective generic and trade names are lamivudine (Epivir), stavudine (Zerit), zalcitabine (Hivid), and didanosine (Videx).

15k. (A)

15l. (E) Fatal and non-fatal cases of pancreatitis, lactic acidosis, and hepatomegaly with steatosis have been reported with the use of nucleoside analogs. Other concerning adverse effects of ddI include retinal changes, optic neuritis, and peripheral neuropathy.

15m. (B) The ddI pediatric powder for oral solution is reconstituted initially with purified water to a concentration of 20 mg/mL and then with an antacid product to a final concentration of 10 mg/mL. The final product should be shaken well before dosing and is stable for 30 days under refrigeration.

15n. (B) The recommended dose of ddI for pediatric patients is 120 mg/m^2 twice daily. For Beverly, this would calculate to 120 mg/m^2 $\times$ 0.85 m^2 = 102 mg or ~ 100 mg twice daily.

15o. (E)

15p. (E)

15q. (B) Zidovudine is a thymidine analog and an inhibitor of the replication of HIV.

15r. (E) Zidovudine therapy may result in granulocytopenia and severe anemia and myopathy. Rare occurrences of lactic acidosis and hepatomegaly have also been reported.

15s. (E)

15t. (C) The recommended initial dose of zidovudine for children aged 3 months to 12 years is 180 mg/m^2 every 6 hours, not to exceed 200 mg per dose.

CASE 16

16a. (C) Nelfinavir is available in 250-mg tablets. Therefore, Kris would need 2 tablets per dose and 6 tablets per day (500 mg = 2 $\times$ 250 mg tabs). For a 30-day supply, she would need 180 tablets (6 tabs/day $\times$ 30 days = 180 tablets).

16b. (A) Lamivudine (Epivir) is known as 3TC. AZT and ddI are known as zidovudine (Retrovir) and didanosine (Videx), respectively.

16c. (A) The respective generic and trade names are stavudine (Zerit), lamivudine (Epivir), zalcitabine (Hivid), and didanosine (Videx).

16d. (B) Stavudine is a synthetic thymidine nucleoside analog that competes with the natural substrate, deoxythymidine triphosphate.

16e. (D) Stavudine is associated with peripheral neuropathy that can be severe and is dose related. Upon discontinuation of therapy, symptoms may worsen temporarily. If resumption of therapy is desired once the symptoms abate, the dose should be adjusted to 50% of the original dose.

16f. (A) The recommended dose of stavudine for patients weighing less than 30 kg is 1 mg/kg every 12 hours. Therefore, Kris should receive 20 mg every 12 hours (1 mg/kg $\times$ 20 kg = 20 mg).

16g. (D) Stavudine is known as d4T while ddI and AZT refer to didanosine and zidovudine, respectively.

16h. (C) Lamivudine is only slightly metabolized with the only known metabolite being a trans-sulfoxide metabolite. Most of the drug is eliminated renally as unchanged drug. Therefore, dosing adjustments are necessary in patients with renal impairment.

16i. (B) Lamivudine is a synthetic nucleoside analog.

16j. (D) The pediatric dose of lamivudine is 4 mg/kg twice a daily up to a maximum of 150 mg twice a day. Therefore, Kris should receive 80 mg po bid (4 mg/kg x 20 kg = 80 mg).

16k. (B) Lamivudine is also marketed as Epivir-HBV and is indicated for the treatment of chronic hepatitis B associated with hepatitis B viral replication and active liver inflammation.

16l. (A)

16m. (C) Both components (lopinavir and ritonavir) of Kaletra are protease inhibitors. Ritonavir inhibits the cytochrome P450-3A mediated metabolism of lopinavir resulting in increased lopinavir serum concentrations. Other drugs metabolized via this same pathway may also be affected by Kaletra necessitating close monitoring of such drug concentrations.

16n. (E) Other adverse effects include elevations of hepatic enzymes, fat redistribution, hemophilia, and gastrointestinal effects (nausea, diarrhea, and abdominal pain).

16o. (B) Kaletra is available in a capsule (lopinavir 133.3 mg/ ritonavir 33.3 mg) and oral solution (lopinavir 80 mg/ritonavir 20 mg/mL) dosage forms. Dosing is based on the lopinavir component. Therefore, Kris is prescribed 200 mg po bid or 400 mg/day; therefore, 80 mg/mL = 400 mg/x; x = 5 mL per day.

16p. (B)

16q. (A) Nelfinavir is also a protease inhibitor and should be discontinued once the combination protease inhibitor product, Kaletra, is initiated.

CASE 17

17a. (C) Type I Diabetes accounts for ~ 10% of the diabetic population and only 15% have a family member with the disease. The main pathological characteristic is an autoimmune destruction of beta cells of the pancreatic Islets of Langerhans in patients with certain homologous leukocyte antibody types. The autoimmune response may also be precipitated by environmental factors such as viruses. Type I patients are prone to ketoacidosis.

17b. (E) Diabetes mellitus is the leading cause of blindness and accounts for ~ 25% of end stage renal failure cases. Neuropathies, as a result of metabolic disturbances in neurons or secondary to microangiopathy, are also a consequence of poorly controlled diabetes.

17c. (B) The diagnosis of diabetes can be made with any combination of two of the following test results: fasting blood glucose > 126 mg/dL, random blood glucose of > 200 mg/dL with hyperglycemic symptoms, or a 2-hour oral glucose tolerance test (OGTT) of more than 200 mg/dL.

17d. (D) A glycosylated hemoglobin (HbA_{1c}) test is recommended as a monitoring parameter for diabetes and reflects an average blood glucose concentration over the past 2–3 months. A value of < 7% is desirable.

17e. (A) Insulin is absorbed more rapidly in the abdomen followed by the upper arm, thigh, and buttocks.

17f. (E) Hypoglycemia may result from excessive insulin dosing. Lipoatrophy is the breakdown of adipose tissue at the insulin injection site. Lipohypertrophy is the result of repeated insulin injections at the same site and may be avoided by rotating injection sites.

17g. (D) Humalog, insulin lispro, is a rapid acting insulin with an onset of action within 15 minutes of dosing. The onset of action of Humulin R, Humulin N, and Ultralente is ~ 0.5, 2, and 4 hours, respectively.

17h. (B)

17i. (D) Humulin R is a clear solution and may be administered subcutaneously or intravenously. It is also available as Humulin 70/30 (Humulin N 70 units and Humulin R 30 units per ml) and Humulin 50/50.

17j. (D) The onset of action of Humulin N is ~ 2–4 hours with a peak effect in ~ 6–10 hours and a duration of ~ 14–24 hours.

17k. (A) The Humulin R should be withdrawn first so that the Humulin R vial does not become contaminated with Humulin N, thus possibly prolonging the onset of action of the Humulin R insulin.

17l. (A) Humulin N insulin is available in a concentration of 100 units/mL. Tricia's morning Humulin N dose is 7 units. Therefore, 100 units/mL = 7 units/x; x = 0.07 mL.

17m. (A) Insulin glargine (Lantus) is a long-acting insulin with a duration of action of at least 24 hours.

17n. (B) Although Lantus has a clear appearance, it is not intended for intravenous administration and should only be given subcutaneously.

17o. (C) Lantus must not be diluted or mixed with other insulins as its pharmacokinetic/pharmacodynamic profile may be altered. Its constant glucose-lowering effect allows for once daily dosing and is thus classified as a long-acting insulin.

17p. (D) Initially, Lantus was only indicated for bedtime administration. However, it is now approved to be given at any time during the day as long as the time is consistent from day to day.

17q. (B) For patients receiving intermediate acting in-sulins on a twice a day schedule, it is recommended to initiate Lantus at a 20% lower dose to decrease the potential risk of hypoglycemia. Since Tricia was receiving Humulin N 10 units/day in divided doses, it would be prudent to initiate Lantus therapy at 8 units/day at bedtime (80% of the Humulin daily dose).

CASE 18

18a. (D) Up to approximately 85% of children that present with Type II diabetes are overweight or obese. Between 45–80% also have at least one parent with diabetes. These children usually present with glycosuria without ketonuria, absent or mild polyuria and polydipsia, and little or no weight loss.

18b. (A) Criteria and guidelines for screening children for diabetes includes: Children overweight plus two additional risks factors (family history, American Indian, African American, Hispanic, Asian/Pacific Islander, signs or conditions associated with insulin resistance), begin screening at age 10 years or onset of puberty, screen every 2 years, and fasting blood glucose test preferred.

18c. (E) The ultimate treatment goal is to decrease the complications associated with diabetes. Normalization of blood glucose concentrations substantially decreases the associated microvascular complications. Other comorbidities such as hypertension and hyperlipidemia should also be controlled.

18d. (A) Lifestyle changes including diet and exercise are essential for patients with diabetes. Successful diabetes management (i.e., fasting blood glucose < 126 mg/dL and HbA1c < 7 %) occurs in fewer than 10% of adult patients without incorporating insulin or oral agents as additional therapy.

18e. (B) The respective generic and trade names are rosiglitazone (Avandia), metformin (Glucophage), acarbose (Precose), and pioglitazone (Actos).

18f. (A) Metformin is a biguanide that not only acts to decrease hepatic glucose output and intestinal absorption of glucose, but also improves insulin sensitivity without a direct effect on pancreatic beta-cell activity. It is recommended as first line therapy for the treatment of Type II diabetes.

18g. (D) One of the major benefits of metformin is that unlike the sulfonylureas, it does not carry the risk of inducing hypoglycemia. Additionally, weight is usually either decreased or remains stable and LDL cholesterol and triglyceride concentrations decrease.

18h. (A) Lactic acidosis is a rare, but highly fatal (~ 50%) complication of metformin therapy that occurs in the face of drug accumulation. Therefore, metformin is contraindicated in patients with impaired renal function.

18i. (B) Metformin is indicated in children ≥ 10 years of age at a starting dose of 500 mg twice a day.

18j. (A) Metformin is also available as a 500-mg extended-release tablet that is indicated for patients ≥ 17 years of age. The usual starting dose is 500 mg once a day.